SKIN
REVOLUTION

Thorsons
An imprint of HarperCollins*Publishers*
1 London Bridge Street
London SE1 9GF

www.harpercollins.co.uk

HarperCollins*Publishers*
1st Floor, Watermarque Building,
Ringsend Road
Dublin 4, Ireland

First published by Thorsons 2022

10 9 8 7 6 5 4 3 2 1

Photography P4 (LH col, 3nd row) 16, 36, 60,
70, 73, 74, 77 (LH col, 2nd and bottom rows
and RH col, 2nd row), 98, 154 (RH col, 3rd row),
158 © Dr Vanita Rattan; P118 Science Photo
Library/Alamy Stock Photo; P154 © Audrey
Fretz on Unsplash (RH col, 3rd row); P225
© Jessica Felicio on Unsplash; P241 © The
Creative Exchange on Unsplash.com (LH col,
3rd row); All other images, Shutterstock.com

Diagram illustrations © Ben Hasler
Design by Studio 7:15

Dr Vanita Rattan asserts the moral right
to be identified as the author of this work

A catalogue record of this book is
available from the British Library

ISBN 978-0-00-847330-3

Printed and bound by GPS Group

SKIN
REVOLUTION

THE ULTIMATE GUIDE TO BEAUTIFUL
AND HEALTHY SKIN OF COLOUR

DR 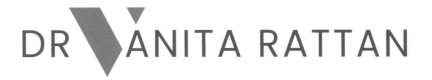 ANITA RATTAN

Thorsons

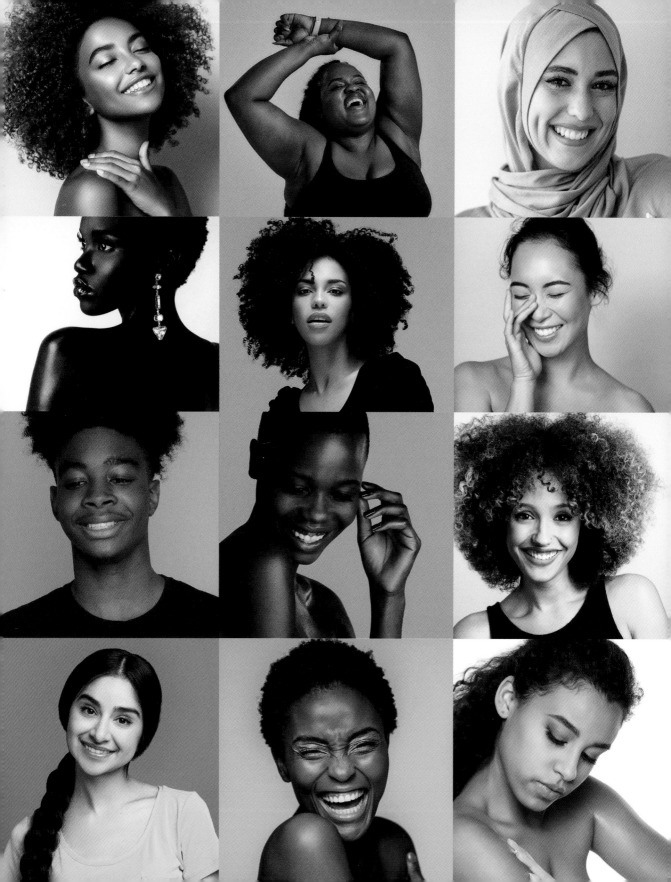

To my skin-of-colour family,

I am honoured and grateful to have been able to serve you.

For those of you who have followed me on social media and have seen my ups and downs firsthand, thank you so much for being my support system. If it wasn't for you, this book could not have been written. You helped me on Instagram with some of the largest polls ever conducted for skin of colour. You helped me choose which chapters to write and even indicated the style in which you wanted the written teaching to be. You allowed me to be open and vulnerable online, which gave me the confidence to reveal so many of my own experiences and faults without feeling embarrassed.

My aim is to empower my global family to buy skincare safely without damaging your skin barrier, to avoid expensive marketing traps and to give our children the correct education about their skin so they have the confidence to live their dreams.

Having investigated hundreds of skincare brands, I was shocked at how little there was for my skin of colour family. It also didn't feel fair that there wasn't enough information for us to be able to educate ourselves. This is why I have dedicated my life to people with skin of colour globally; to ensure you have the best skin of your lives and you don't waste your hard-earned money on ineffective products.

I've worked extremely hard on this book to make it the number one resource for men, women and children with skin of colour across the world. I hope you find it useful and that I made you proud. As you know, I have never accepted sponsorship and I never will – honest research and education is my love letter to my skin of colour family.

I promise I will continue to research, educate and do the best I can for all of us. All my love always, Dr V xxx

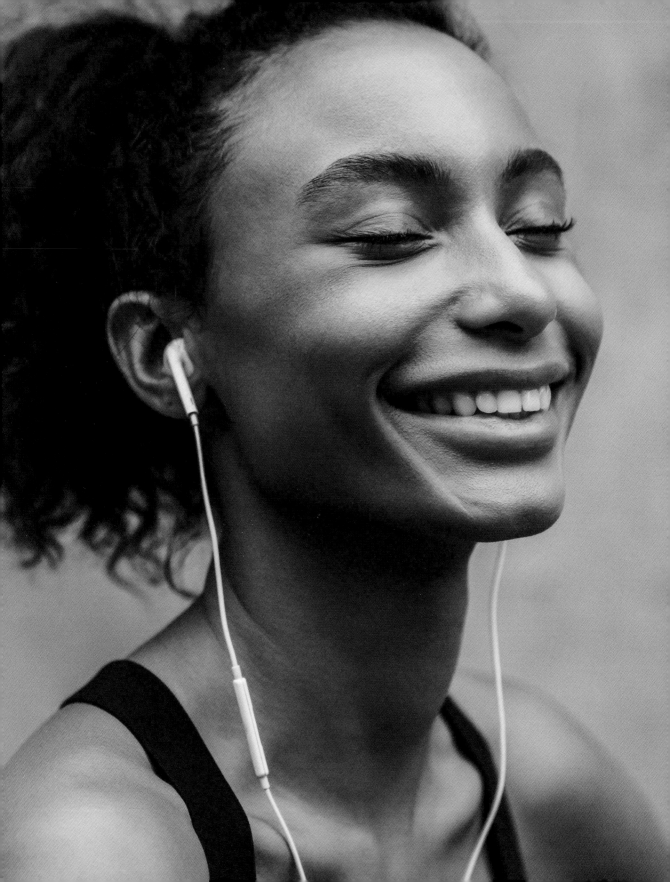

'Understanding the complexities of skin of colour is both a science and an art. Dr Vanita has managed to make a very difficult subject easy, fun and enjoyable to learn in this labour of love. I am so excited for all of the enthusiasm and inspiration this book will create in young skin of colour future physicians, scientists and entrepreneurs.'

Dr Alexis Stephens DO, FAOCD, FAAD

Founder and CEO of Parkland Dermatology, Award-winning Board Certified Dermatologist, Beauty Chemist, Cosmetic, Medical and Skin of Colour Expert

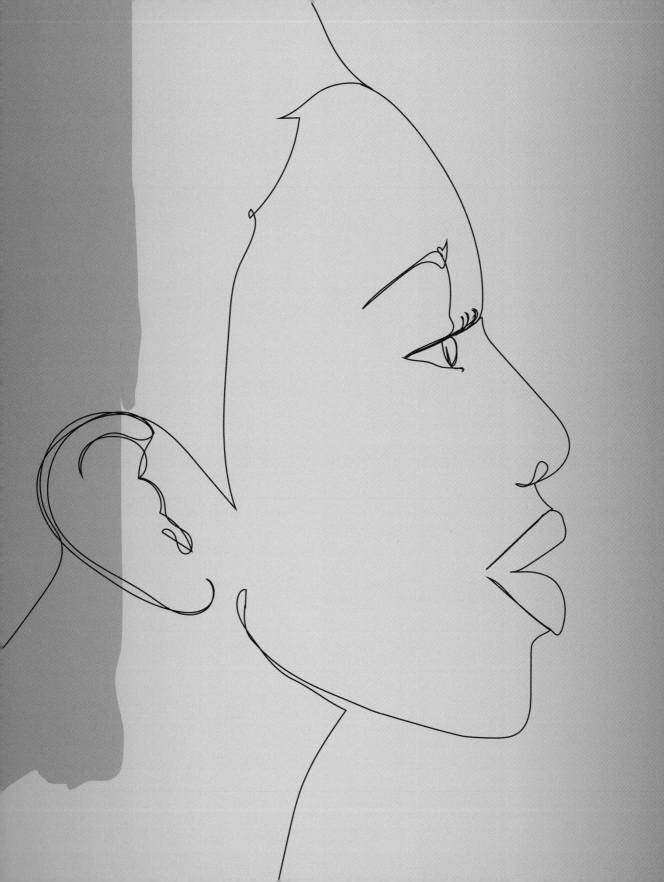

CONTENTS

OUR MELANIN-RICH SKIN IS BEAUTIFUL AND SHOULD BE TREATED THAT WAY.

Introduction

Welcome to our Skin Revolution. I hope that this book will radically transform your approach to skincare by providing you with the tools to decipher the ingredients within products, discount the marketing hype on the packaging, demystify your skin's chemistry and empower you to do right by your skin throughout your lifetime.

Approximately 5 in 7 people in the world have skin of colour. We are a global majority.

Despite this figure, five-sevenths of skincare products do not cater to skin of colour. In fact, we struggle to find products suitable for our skin. I have analysed over 150 brands for my unsponsored YouTube channel to decode the ingredients list and let you know if the product being reviewed is suitable for us or not. So far my channel has had 30 million views in just one year, with requests for me to test new products coming in from viewers all the time, which shows just how much this information is needed – and how hard it is to find.

Skin Revolution has one mission at its heart: to provide much-needed tender loving care to the skin of colour community.

It is no secret that our skin shades are underrepresented in beauty and fashion, but our melanin-rich skin is beautiful and should be treated as such.

This book is the result of over a decade of study and research that I have undertaken in the formulation of skincare products specifically for skin of colour. This information took hundreds of thousands of pounds in research and failed clinical trials. It has cost me many sleepless nights, which has felt lonely at times. However, out of that pain and frustration I identified the most effective ingredients for skin of colour, the correct percentages and how to combine them so that our global skin of colour family receives the best for our skin. Although some people have asked if I am completely sure I want to share my insider secrets from making these products – in case they are used by cosmetics competitors – I have never been more certain in my response: 100 per cent, yes.

I am here to serve my skin of colour family – you, the readers of this book – across the world. I hope to present you with education and empowerment about the choices you are making for your skin. By lifting the curtain on the skincare industry, I'm handing back power to you, the consumer. This is the reason why I started my YouTube channel in 2019: Dr Vanita Rattan – Dedicated to Skin of Colour.

The information in this book is my answer to the hundreds of queries sent in by followers of my channel, who want to better understand how to take care of their melanin-rich skin.

Skincare products can sometimes be mystifying and overwhelming, with product promises, patch tests, timelines for visible results and an infinite array of creams, gels, oils and toners on offer.

> *I'm here to help you on your skincare journey, whether you're just starting out or are already deep into a daily ten-step skincare routine.*

The sheer array of products and competing claims makes it easier for cosmetics companies to dazzle you into buying products, but remember that the beautiful photoshoot images have zero to do with what is in the bottle.

Throughout these chapters I have included my own formulation insights to show how skincare products are made and shared what I have learned throughout my journey as a cosmetic formulator. By the end of this book you should be able to tell me what active ingredients you want to see in your skincare products to solve a particular problem and have a confident understanding of how to look after your unique and beautiful skin.

I first began my journey in cosmetic formulation dedicated solely to skin of colour about twelve years ago. Back then, there was much we were yet to discover. It wasn't common knowledge that our melanocytes (the melanin-producing cells in our skin) were more reactive and unpredictable than in Caucasian skin.

> *Hyperpigmentation is the number one skin concern for skin of colour.*

Put simply, this is when melanin production increases in a specific area. Hyperpigmentation leads to dark patches on the skin, which can be distressing and restrictive for what you wear. It can happen on the face from acne, a scar or as melasma from UV radiation. It can occur during puberty – usually affecting the underarms, inner thighs, knees and around the mouth. It can appear after any inflammation from a rash, eczema, insect bite or a cut. This means we need to know how to prevent it in the first place and how to treat it quickly to get the best results.

Skin of colour needs different treatments and ingredient concentrations than Caucasian skin. In the past, we were completely reliant on product marketing messages, even if the ingredients didn't match up with the claims, which left us confused and with unsatisfying results. And even though doctors knew the side-effect of hyperpigmentation treatments was often *more* hyperpigmentation, they were completely reliant on cosmetic companies to resolve those issues for skin of colour.

Now, the picture is different. The word is spreading fast that skin of colour requires products that are designed specifically for our issues and that won't cause unnecessary irritation. I want us to become empowered in our skincare choices, together. One follower of my channel, who is living in Jamaica, let me know that she had been browsing in the cosmetics aisle of a store and had come across another skin-of-colour sister doing the exact same thing. After a brief exchange, they realised that they were both following the advice I had shared on my Instagram page. Not only did this warm my heart, it showed me how we are learning to read ingredients lists to see if products are actually able to do what they claim, and that this movement is truly global.

Newer platforms like TikTok mean that information and education on skincare is being introduced to the next generation at a much younger age. These platforms can provide young people with information that will help them avoid causing harm to their skin that would normally only be available from a specialist doctor or aesthetic practitioner – although be warned that they can also introduce worrying misinformation (more on that later!). I wanted to write this book so that it could be used as a tool for people of any age, at any point in their skincare journey, to learn how to look after their body's biggest organ. At last, skin of colour is rightly being recognised as a priority, so much so that I am being approached by brands globally to assist with formulas for skin of colour to make products suitable for us. This would have been unthinkable only a few years ago.

> *As a formulator with a line of products created for skin of colour, I often get asked why such skincare products have not been made by any big manufacturers yet.*

My critics might argue that big companies are surely more equipped than I am to research and create for skin of colour. While larger companies certainly have the resources to mass-produce at a cheaper price than I can, and no doubt have more extensive research facilities, the problem stems from not knowing that skin of colour requires products that cater for our skin. You only know there is a problem in the skincare offering if you have skin of colour and realise products on the shelf aren't working or are making the situation worse. A common example is if you have hyperpigmentation, have tried to treat it, then realised the product you bought was burning your skin and making the problem worse.

The gap in the market for skin of colour exists for three main reasons:

- You need to BE the demographic to know there is a problem.
- It is not enough to just BE the demographic, you need to know how to formulate and conduct trials for skin of colour, which requires an immense amount of knowledge and skill.
- Cosmetic companies need to know if a venture is financially viable before embarking on years of costly research. As they have never considered the gap in product experience for those with skin of colour, they have not been keen to commit resources to creating bespoke skincare.

It's time to bridge the gap between research on skin of colour and the manufacturing of skincare products.

My critics might ask me, 'What makes you think you are so special that nobody else has figured this all out?' To which my response is that I am really nothing special at all. All I have is my unwavering commitment to do the best by skin of colour, a mission helped by the fact that I am a workaholic who loves to tackle problems that no one else has tried to and I won't stop until I have succeeded. I am the child of immigrants, and if any of you have the same background you will know that failure is never an option and an immense work ethic, bordering on obsession, is the norm. My parents owned a cosmetics company and so I got to experiment in their lab with their ingredients and their cosmetic formulator. I was also fortunate that I had two degrees – a Medical Degree (MBBS) and a (BSc) in Physiology and Pharmacology.

It is quite rare for a doctor to not work in a hospital after six years of medical school. To deviate from practising medicine face-to-face with patients and instead venture into a lab to learn how to 'make creams' is not really on the cards when you feel that you could be saving lives! But I knew that this journey was important because the needs of the skin of colour community had not yet been met by mainstream cosmetics companies.

Being both a doctor and a cosmetic formulator gives me a unique understanding of how ingredients should be combined and how the resulting products affect people in a clinical setting. It also helped me to read clinical trials, which confirmed the gaping holes in research for skin of colour aesthetics.

Do you feel your local drugstore/pharmacy caters for skin of colour sufficiently?

Yes (362 responses)   **No** (3378 responses)

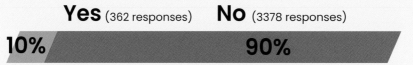

10%   90%

Have you burnt, had a reaction, damaged your skin barrier or got more pigmentation using cosmetic cream from your local drugstore/pharmacy?

Yes (2202 responses)   **No** (934 responses)

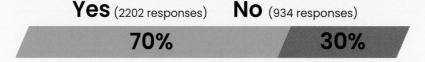

70%   30%

Do you wish there was an affordable skin of colour line with no fragrance, denatured alcohol or essential oils?

Yes (4385 responses)   **No** (160 responses)

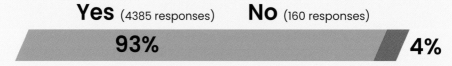

93%   4%

Note: Throughout this book you will see polls conducted on my Instagram specifically for skin of colour. Each poll received thousands of responses, making them some of the largest ever conducted on skincare for S.O.C.

What is INCI?

International Nomenclature of Cosmetic Ingredients

This is the list of internationally uniform names for identifying cosmetic ingredients. There are over 16,000 ingredients in the INCI database.

There is a disconnect between the worlds of clinical study and cosmetic formulation. This may help to explain why we do not have more research in this area. And it also helps to explain why I was able to be the bridge between this research and the products that are made for skin of colour. Sometimes the cosmetic formulator will read their literature from the ingredient supplier and won't know how it impacts the patient in a clinical setting. The doctor, on the other hand, has not been taught to read INCI lists and is reliant on marketing and company reps, as understanding how ingredients in cosmetic products work is not a subject that is taught at medical school.

Join the Dr V S.O.C Family on Facebook

So many people are joining our skin-of-colour family, and you can get started on this journey, too. All you need to be is:

- **Someone who has watched over 10 Dr Vanita Rattan YouTube videos and can decode half their skincare ingredients list.**

- **A scientific, logical thinker.**

- **Someone who shares the information with loved ones so they can see through marketing and not waste money on products that are either ineffective or, worse, damage the skin barrier.**

- **Someone with the healthiest skin they have ever experienced.**

- **Someone who has an improved relationship and understanding of their skin, giving them confidence and empowerment.**

By reading this book, you're already on your first steps to joining the Dr V's S.O.C family! And if you've already joined our community of education and empowerment, then you know who you are!

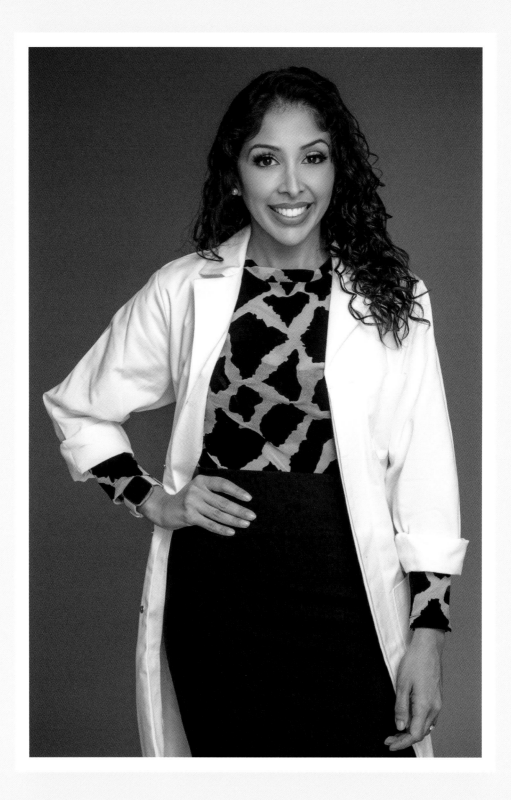

I made it my mission to conduct clinical studies to discover the ingredients and percentages that are suitable for skin of colour. In the process, every kit I made was – and still is – given to a cohort of people with skin of colour for independent clinical studies to assess the success rates of the products but also the risk of irritation and hyperpigmentation. I hope more brands start doing this kind of research as part of their formulation process because it is really important to understand that while individual ingredients work well, they may not work well in combination – specifically for skin of colour. Our skin cannot tolerate too much inflammation, and this is one of the reasons why creating cocktail creams is difficult for skin of colour.

The future of skin of colour

Skin of colour has historically been ignored by mainstream cosmetics companies (I'm sure you remember the excitement and buzz around the nuanced array of colour-match foundation for skin of colour when Fenty Beauty launched!). So, what's next? I predict that more products will be released that say 'for skin of colour' on the packaging as the cosmetics industry finally wakes up to the huge demand for these products. However, it is up to you to analyse the ingredients because anyone can write 'for skin of colour' on their packaging. At the moment it is an unregulated term. That's why this book has a comprehensive ingredients section as well as advice on which ingredients to use for particular skin conditions or concerns, as well as how to layer and use them to treat multiple skin conditions. Beyond this, my YouTube channel will be a complete reference library of which products (old and new) I recommend and which ones I would avoid.

I think the next generation will start to take care of their skin from a younger age. And with increased knowledge they will also experience fewer burns, less hyperpigmentation and be able to preserve their youthfulness for longer.

As a cosmetic formulator, I hope we will get an international rating for the sustainability of ingredients and a carbon footprint rating for both ingredients and packaging so we can produce products that are safe for our planet as well as for future generations.

The Skin Revolution starts here

Great skin makes you feel great – it's a simple and timeless truth. This book is my love letter to our skin of colour family around the world. This book is for us – and for future generations – because our melanin deserves the very best!

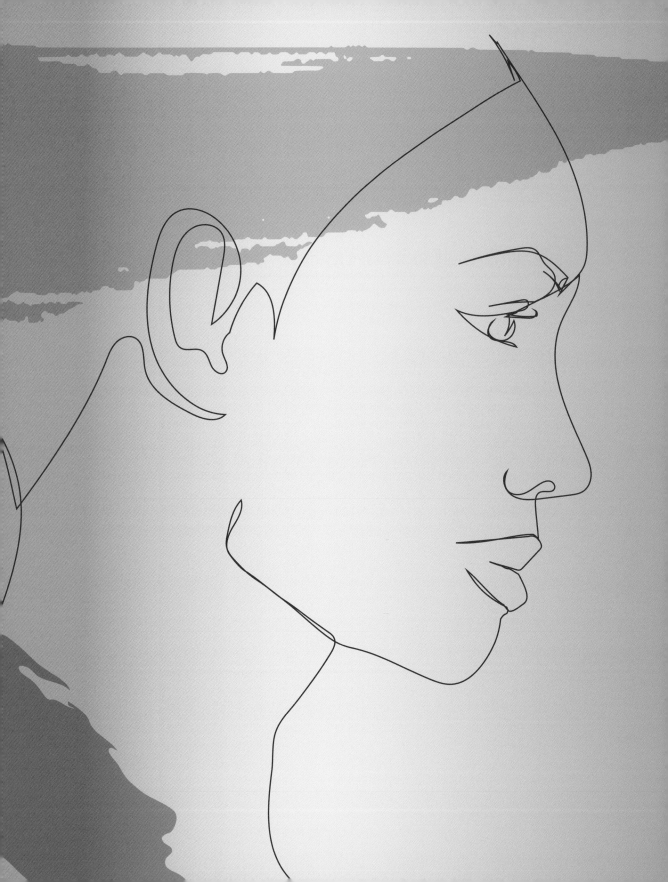

1

Getting to know your

SKIN

Is it really that important for us to understand the science of skin, or can I skip this chapter and just jump ahead to find out what routine I should follow for my combination skin?

The answer is ... this is an ESSENTIAL chapter. My aim here is to explain the different layers that make up your skin, the role of melanin, how ingredients work on these layers and outline the classic mistakes that most people make so that you can avoid them! If you don't understand skin anatomy and physiology, you won't know how ingredients and products actually work. If you don't know how products and ingredients work, you will continue to fall for all the marketing gimmicks, expensive adverts or enchanting-smelling creams that are vying for your attention – and money.

I want to empower you to make the right choices by giving you the knowledge and science to truly understand your skin, pay attention to it closely and learn how it recovers and renews itself each cell cycle, depending on your age, skin type and skin concerns.

The science that follows will help you to understand your skin from the tiniest skin cell all the way up to the biggest pore that you wish you could minimise!

Being confident in your own skin is everything.

Everyone wants to get that glow – the healthy, radiant skin that makes them feel amazing every day. We all want to feel comfortable in our skin and give it the love and care it needs in order to look and feel as good as possible.

The first impression we usually have of a person is from their face. We can instantly estimate age and health and assess if someone might be stressed or if they haven't been sleeping well.

The skin performs major functions to keep our bodies healthy, too, such as keeping bacteria out, performing thermoregulation (the body's process for regulating your body temperature) and keeping our internal structures intact. But for the purposes of this book we will focus more on practical step-by-step information to help you understand how to care for your skin, stop wasting money and avoid irritation to your body's largest organ!

This journey through our skin is your roadmap to understanding how different ingredients work – and where they work or have an effect in our skin – so here's a bit of science before we start to help you get to know your skin.

The layers of the skin and why they are important

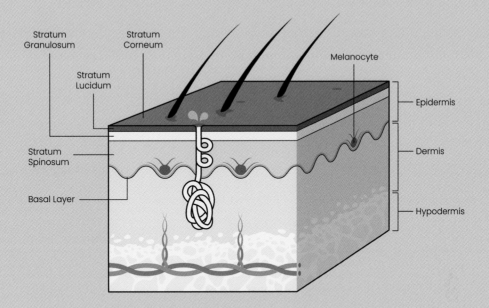

Stratum Granulosum
Stratum Corneum
Stratum Lucidum
Melanocyte
Epidermis
Stratum Spinosum
Dermis
Basal Layer
Hypodermis

Hypodermis – this is the deepest skin layer, primarily made of fat, which is located under the dermis. This layer acts as a cushion to protect all our organs – liver, heart, kidneys as well as muscle and bones – against shocks and knocks and also aids temperature insulation. As we age, we lose fat in these areas, which causes the skin to shrink. This is why losing a lot of weight after the age of 40 years old can mean your skin is less elastic and doesn't bounce back into place like it used to in our youth.

Dermis – above the hypodermis sits the dermis. This is the middle layer of skin, which is about 2mm thick. Visually, imagine a mesh of collagen and elastin, for strength and elasticity, forming the scaffolding of the skin. Peak collagen is at 21 years old, then after this we produce 1 per cent less collagen annually. This leads to sagging skin and fine lines from your mid to late twenties, which is why using SPF50 from a young age is important. (I will go into more details about anti-ageing skincare through the decades in chapter five.)

Now imagine this meshwork of collagen and elastin are soaked in water magnets called glycosaminoglycans (a common one that you might have heard of is hyaluronic acid). Their purpose is to bind water molecules, which keeps the dermis hydrated and plump.

Also among the collagen/elastin mesh and the water-binding glycosaminoglycans you have an immune system that responds to stimuli, leading to inflammation triggering your melanocytes (melanin-producing cells), which in turn leads to hyperpigmentation (see chapter four). This inflammatory cascade is complex and not well understood, but what we do know is we need to minimise any trigger of inflammation to minimise chances of PIH (Post-inflammatory Hyperpigmentation).

> *Keeping our skin calm and happy is essential for skin of colour, in order to avoid hyperpigmentation.*

Blood vessels constrict and dilate to control body temperature, which is why your skin turns red or deepens in shade after exercising. The blood vessels are bringing oxygen to the dermis to regulate your temperature, as well as to bring nutrients to cells and remove carbon dioxide. However, there are no blood vessels in the epidermis.

> *But if there are no blood vessels in our dermis, does that mean the top layer of skin is basically dead skin cells?*

The border between the epidermis and the dermis is a wavy line called the dermal-epidermal junction (science is not known for its imaginative names!). This wavy dermal-epidermal junction (where the epidermis and dermis meet, also known as the basal layer) creates a large surface area where the transfer of nutrients and oxygen to the lower levels of the epidermis can take place. The upper layers of the epidermis are indeed dead. This is important to know because exfoliation for skin of colour should only remove dead skin cells through controlled chemical exfoliation (see chapter two on exfoliation, pages 40–1) not aggressive physical exfoliation, which can remove live epidermal cells, which can lead to inflammation and sensitivity.

As you age, this wavy junction between the dermis and epidermis flattens, which means there is a smaller surface area for oxygen and nutrient transfer. This is one of the reasons for skin ageing.

> **Epidermis –** this is where almost all the magic happens with cosmetic creams. The key point is that the epidermis is constantly turning over and shedding; new skin cells start at the basal layer and travel up the skin conveyor belt until they are seen on the surface. This process is called **cell renewal.**

> *The epidermis is 0.1 mm thick, on average, which is the same thickness as the pages in this book!*

How melanin is produced

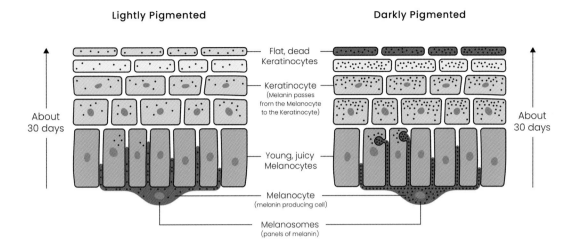

| Lightly Pigmented | | Darkly Pigmented |

Flat, dead Keratinocytes

Keratinocyte
(Melanin passes from the Melanocyte to the Keratinocyte)

About 30 days

Young, juicy Melanocytes

Melanocyte
(melanin producing cell)

Melanosomes
(panels of melanin)

Skincare science

So now let's get a bit deeper into the science, because understanding the properties of skin and how it changes as we age will help you understand why it behaves the way it does and how you can best take care of it.

Cell renewal slows drastically as we age

This means that as we age we should expect progressively more:

- wrinkles
- hyperpigmentation
- dull skin
- poor penetration of active ingredients

The good news is that there are ways in which you can increase cell turnover and improve skin structure, and we will cover these in the anti-ageing chapter (see chapter five).

Our beautiful melanin acts as a partial shield to UV rays, which is why we don't burn as quickly.

Melanocytes live at the basal layer, on the wavy line between the dermis and epidermis. They look like octopuses because they have several arms, and they produce parcels of melanin called melanosomes that pass to surrounding skin cells (keratinocytes). These cells pass up the skin conveyor belt to the surface, where pigment is seen. People with skin of colour have more melanin, which gives better UV protection.

MYTH: Skin of colour has more melanocytes than Caucasian skin

TRUTH: We all have one melanocyte for about 36 keratinocytes. However, melanocytes in darker skins are bigger, the parcels of pigment (melanosomes) are larger and there are more of them per melanocyte. In addition, the melanocytes are easier to activate in skin of colour. There are different types of melanin, too, and skin of colour has also relatively more 'brown' eumelanin compared to 'light-red' pheomelanin.

The skin is considered waxy and waterproof, which makes it hard for cosmetic creams and active ingredients to penetrate it to get to the layers below.

Skin cells are held together by protein links called corneodesmosomes. These are surrounded by lipids (ceramides, fatty acids and cholesterol) that maintain the skin barrier, reducing the evaporation of water from the skin (known as transepidermal water loss, or TEWL). It is important to hydrate the skin, because when it is dehydrated it looks dull, loses the ability to plump up rapidly and tends to be more sensitive to ingredients, which can then lead to more reactions. This barrier is also essential to keep out irritants such as bacteria, fungi and chemicals.

Can you guess what happens if this barrier is out of balance? You will experience some, or most if you're unlucky, of these symptoms:

- Red, burgundy or deep-purple areas of inflammation
- Dryness
- Itching
- Bleeding (sometimes)

This can progress to an eczematous type of reaction and a secondary infection.

Did you know the skin's moisture barrier is actually slightly acidic and has a pH of 4.5 to 6?

This is called the acid mantle and is made by secretions from sweat and sebaceous glands. The pH of skin of colour is the same as for Caucasian skin.

Why using soap is not a good idea

Alkaline soaps (with a pH higher than 7), such as bar soaps, can disrupt the acid environment of the skin as well as the keratin in skin, which allows irritants to enter the skin and encourages water to evaporate from it.

pH level of skin

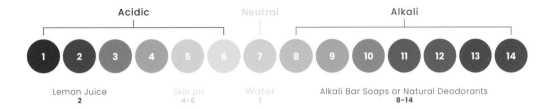

So why is the skin acidic? It is for a number of reasons, all of which support the skin's health:

- It stops the growth of microorganisms, including bacteria and fungi.
- It helps keep keratin proteins hard and maintains the integrity of the skin. This means the proteins are held together tightly, but if the pH level rises the keratin protein softens and the skin barrier becomes compromised, which allows irritants to enter.

Pores, sweat and sebum

'Acne breakouts get me really down.'
'I hate my large pores.'
'How do I stop my armpits from sweating?'

Have you ever looked at a huge open pore in the mirror and wondered what you can do to make it smaller, then wondered why it's there at all? Let's get into why this happens by first understanding the links between pores, sweat and breakouts.

Pores are where the epidermis dips and falls into the dermis to create an opening to the surface, and sweat glands and sebaceous glands are connected to the pore. Just like a well brings water to the surface, a pore brings sebum and sweat to the surface.

There are a few reasons why sweat and sebum are important for your skin:

Thermoregulation – when you or the weather are hot, sweat is released, which helps to cool the skin surface as it is evaporated, taking heat with it. When it is cold, sebum contains more lipids to protect against heat loss via evaporation.

Moisture barrier – a barrier at the skin surface is essential because it holds in moisture, which keeps the epidermis hydrated. Squalene is present in sebum, and is an emollient and antioxidant. This is why I like to use Squalane (the stable form of squalene) in skincare for skin of colour, as it is skin-identical.

Microorganisms – the acidic moisture barrier will keep bacteria and fungi at bay. This is why we do not want to raise the pH of our skin by using high-pH ingredients on it.

How are pores involved in breakouts?

The base of your pores is constantly shedding skin cells. You now have a delicious soup of fatty sebum and skin cells (keratinocytes), which can form a plug and lead to enlarged pores or acne.

Can you guess where the sebaceous glands are mainly located?

Scalp
Face
Chest
Back

In other words, all of these are problem areas where acne breakouts occur.

Do you have skin of colour?

'I'm a fair-skinned Asian, do I have skin of colour?'
'I'm olive toned; do I have skin of colour?'

Skin of colour is melanin-rich black and brown skin. Most people of colour have skin of colour, however, this can be in various shades, with different tones and undertones (cool, warm, neutral or a mix of these). Because of this variation in colour, I have been asked the above questions before, by people trying to understand their own skin tone.

Rule of thumb:

If you are more likely to tan rather than burn in the sun, you are considered to have **skin of colour.**

The reason you are more likely to tan is because your melanocytes (melanin-producing cells) are easier to trigger. In addition, you are more likely to suffer from hyperpigmentation.

As I have said on my YouTube channel countless times, skin of colour needs particular care:

'One scratch, one bite or one burn and we hyperpigment.'

The **Fitzpatrick Scale** can help here, too.

Developed in 1975 by a white American dermatologist, originally to assess the risk of skin cancer, this scale classifies skin according to how much melanin it contains and how it responds to UV radiation. Many people may find they are in between skin types. This scale is intended as a guide to help you identify your own skin type.

	Type 1	Type 2	Type 3	Type 4	Type 5	Type 6
Skin Colour	Very light, pale white	Fair, white	Medium white to olive/ golden	Olive, moderate brown	Dark brown	Very dark brown/ black
Eye Colour	Blue/green	Blue/green	Light brown	Light brown/ dark brown	Dark brown	Dark brown
Hair Colour	Red/ blonde	Blonde	Dark brown	Dark brown	Dark brown	Dark brown/ black
Skin In Sun	Always burns/ never tans/ freckles present	Usually burns/tans with much difficulty	Mild burn/ gradual tan	Rarely burns/ easily tans	Hard to burn/ always tans	Never burns/ tans easily

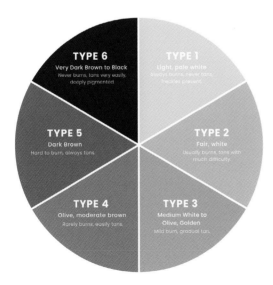

Which Fitzpatrick Scale category is considered skin of colour?

Types 4, 5 and 6 are clear cut and it's easy to see these are skin of colour. Those with type 3 may or may not identify themselves as people of colour, but it's important to recognise that these people also are prone to hyperpigmentation and have skin of colour. They are more likely to tan rather than burn in the sun, because they are rich in melanin, the pigment that gives our skin its colour.

NO ONE KNOWS YOUR SKIN BETTER THAN YOU, BUT A LITTLE SCIENCE CAN HELP YOU TAKE BETTER CARE OF IT.

You'll notice that 1 and 2 of the 6 Fitzpatrick types focus on what we might typically call 'white' skin. This is reflective of the disproportionate focus on white skin in dermatology, and the biases against dark skin tones in most of recent history. As recently as 2018, a study of more than 4,000 images in four major US medical textbooks found only 4.5% of images showed dark skin.

Did you also know that the emojis we use to communicate with each other every day are actually based on the Fitzpatrick Scale? If you've ever been dissatisfied by the lack of range of darker skin tones to send your thumbs-up to a friend, this is why! Skin of colour is incredibly diverse in the range of shades and tones produced by different types and concentrations of melanin – and it's important to know what the richness of melanin in our skin means for our skincare.

Skin of colour needs special care

Darker skin tends to be slightly drier, especially as we age.

There is slightly higher transepidermal water loss (see page 24) in darker skin, which means that dark skin is often drier. This could be due to the lower ceramide level in the top layer of the epidermis (the stratum corneum). Ceramides are fats naturally found in the top layers of skin between cells, which improve the function of the skin barrier by holding water in the skin.

This is why these ingredients are essential in a moisturiser:
- ceramides (needs to be in airless pump for stability)
- amino acids (peptides)
- humectants

Skin of colour must avoid irritating ingredients and procedures. The Fitzpatrick Scale of 4 to 6 have increased sensitivity to irritants but show less erythema (redness/burgundy colour area). This means that irritation is not always immediately visible as erythema in skin of colour, so we need to be extra careful to avoid irritating our skin. I always recommend avoiding:

- Drying alcohols
- Essential oils
- Fragrance
- Applying two irritating ingredients together, such as glycolic acid and retinol (see page 107)

Skin of colour doesn't wrinkle as fast as skin tones from the Fitzpatrick Scale 1 and 2 because in the dermis, cells that produce collagen and elastin are larger, collagen bundles are smaller, packed tighter and more parallel to the epidermis compared to lighter skin.

The two points above, in combination with more sun protection from melanin, means skin of colour doesn't wrinkle as fast as Caucasian skin. However...

This is not licence for you to stop wearing your SPF50!

Skin of colour is prone to melasma if not protected against UVA and UVB. (See page 66 on how to choose the best sunscreen.)

So, it's important before we get too far into this book to make a few decisions about your skin and skincare. To help to do this, ask yourself these questions:

Which Fitzpatrick skin type are you?

Do you have skin of colour?

Do you use amino acids, ceramides and hyaluronic acids in your moisturiser?

Do you wear SPF50? Is it mineral or chemical? (more about this later)

Identifying your skin type

You will have most definitely heard talk about skin types before, whether it's on the label of a cleanser designed to tackle oily skin, or a cream for very dry skin. But what are skin types, and how do they help us with our skincare regime? Here are the three main skin types that are defined on product labels, and their specific characteristics:

Dry Skin
Skin feels tight and uncomfortable. It is often sensitive because the skin barrier may be compromised and it can appear dull.

Combination Skin
Skin is often drier on the cheeks and oilier on the T-zone – the area across the forehead and nose.

Oily Skin
After a few hours of washing your face, your skin looks and feels shiny.

Normal Skin
You are one of the lucky ones. Your skin doesn't feel tight or dry after washing it, even if you don't wear moisturiser. In fact, you probably are the last skin type to look at skincare, as it has never been a problem for you or caused you any reason

to feel insecure. The downside may be that the lack of skincare education may mean less sunscreen usage and earlier pigmentation. With normal skin, just wear moisturiser and SPF50 from childhood onwards until you need to add in more actives.

Here are a few of the most common questions I get asked about skin types:

How does skin of colour relate to skin types – for instance, does melanin affect skin type?

Melanin does NOT affect skin type. You can have skin of colour and still have any of the four classic skin types – dry, oily, combination or normal. Although skin of colour has fewer ceramides than Caucasian skin, it can still be oily or normal.

Does your skin type ever change throughout your lifetime, for instance, you have combination skin that becomes dry skin when you're older?

Yes, your skin is likely to change with time. It is likely to be normal or dry (with eczema) in youth, oily as a teen, fluctuate during your menstruation cycle, then become dry during menopause – and in old age for both men and women.

What are the limitations of this skin-type labelling system, if any?

The fact that your skin can move between the different types quite quickly can be confusing, because suddenly the skincare you have been using for years is no longer effective. This is why it is important to pay attention to your skin and to internal/external triggers. For example, stress can trigger acne, Hormone Replacement Therapy (HRT) or the Pill can trigger melasma, and alcohol can dehydrate the skin and make pores appear bigger.

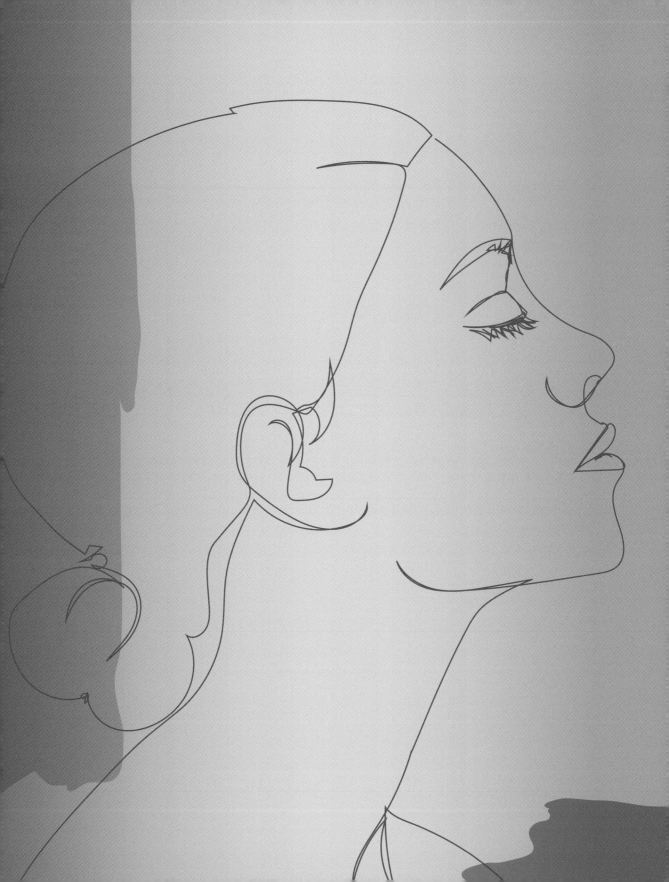

2

Getting savvy with looking after your

SKIN

So now you have identified your skin type, let's get to the good stuff – what we are all here for. What are the best products for your skin, and how can you avoid the ones that will do you no good at all, or even cause you harm?

The most common false or unregulated marketing terms

The reason I started my YouTube channel was to go through cosmetic ingredient lists to show whether or not the ingredients matched with the marketing claims and to share my findings. At the time of writing, I have reviewed over 150 global brands, and here are some of my more shocking discoveries:

Non-comedogenic – a label may indicate that it won't clog the pores. However, this is an unregulated term, and in fact I struggle to find a non-comedogenic cream without comedogenic ingredients. I agree that whether a cream is comedogenic or non-comedogenic is not just about ingredients, it is also the percentage and formulation process, but when the goal is to create a non-comedogenic moisturiser for acne-prone skin your mind should start thinking of humectants that will work well in a gel. You may add sebum-controlling niacinamide or skin-soothing aloe vera. We no longer test if a product is comedogenic on animals in the EU and UK (thank goodness!), so there is no strict threshold for comedogenic versus non-comedogenic product status. It is good to know which ingredients you may want to avoid, such as coconut oil, shea butter, petroleum or petrolatum, so you can read the cosmetic ingredients list with confidence and deduce if the product is good for your skin or not.

Animal testing of cosmetics was banned:

In the UK in 1998
Across the EU in 2013
The legislation is part of EU Regulation 1223/2009 (Cosmetics Regulation)

Maximum strength or professional strength – again, this doesn't mean anything, it just gives the impression that the product is the best. Is it trying to suggest the product is doctor approved or made by a doctor? Even if it is manufactured by a doctor, this fact has no bearing on the percentage of active ingredients used when it comes to cosmetics.

Doctor-owned brands – this will come as a shock to you, as my own brand has been formulated by a doctor … me! However, just because a brand is owned or endorsed by a doctor should not sway you to buy it.

I have reviewed far too many doctor own-brands that are loaded with irritants and active ingredients well below the therapeutic range just so it can be put on packaging. This can legitimately happen as there is no regulation to enforce whether the ingredients used are at the ideal percentages.

Anti-ageing – another unregulated term. I was shocked when I investigated a well-known pharmacy brand and read that the ingredients of the bestselling anti-ageing cream had zero active ingredients to boost collagen, no antioxidants and no skin-replenishing ceramides or peptides. It was just a basic moisturiser with fragrance that was actually more likely to lead to ageing if the consumer got contact dermatitis from it. This will never happen to you, though! (Please read chapter three on Ingredients.)

Natural – another unregulated term. 'Natural' is often used to describe skincare that includes ingredients found in nature (for example, aloe vera or shea butter) and that are not synthetic. However, it's another unregulated term that has no clear definition when it is used to describe skincare products and doesn't specify how those ingredients are formulated in the final product. For example, natural ingredients often need to be synthesised to be useful in a product (see page 112).

Chemical-free – there is no such thing as chemical-free skincare: even water is a chemical – H_2O. You see how easy it is to use marketing to dupe the public?

Hypoallergenic – another unregulated term, one that I've been tricked by before! I bought a body wash that I assumed would be gentler on my skin as it had 'hypoallergenic' written on a white, medical-looking (boring, therefore trustworthy) package. However, it was only once I was in the shower and reading through the list of ingredients that I saw the sixth ingredient was fragrance. Fragrance is the number one cause of contact dermatitis (when skin becomes inflamed after contact with an allergen or irritant). I share this so you can learn from my mistake and *always read the label*!

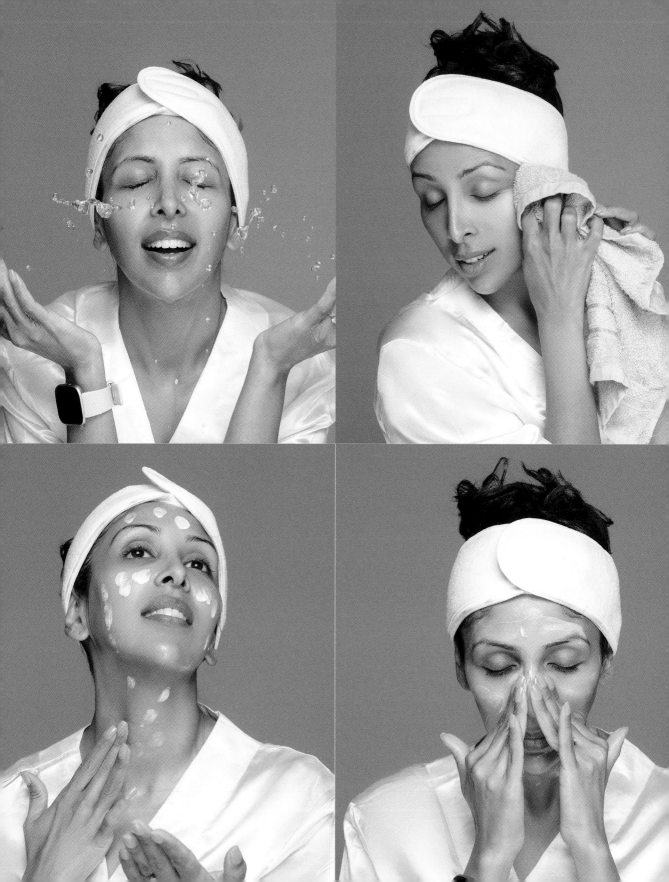

Establishing a basic skincare routine

Looking after your skin is more complicated than just cleansing and moisturising, and it's important to develop a daily routine that is tailored for your skin's needs.

This is a basic five-step skincare routine for skincare beginners as well as seasoned skincare aficionados. It can be adapted to suit your individual skin's needs – whether that's anti-ageing, or treating specific skin conditions such as melasma, or a combination of skin concerns (see the relevant chapters for specific skin issues).

A classic mistake that people make when starting a skincare routine is that they get bored after a week of not seeing results and think it is not working, so they stop. The reason why you should stick with a routine for at least three months is because one cell cycle is about 30–40 days long, and you would need to complete 2–3 cell cycles to determine the effectiveness of your product. If you don't do this you have wasted your money, and if you start adding more and more actives to see 'faster' results it may lead to breakouts and pigmentation. So have patience and stick with your routine for three months. And don't worry about making mistakes – I've got you! You'll see the classic mistakes made at each step, so you can be prepared.

Step-by-step daily routine

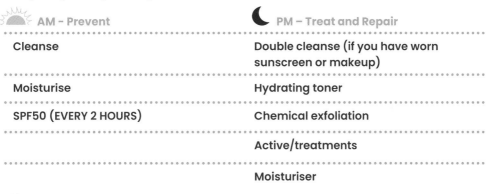

☀ AM - Prevent	🌙 PM – Treat and Repair
Cleanse	Double cleanse (if you have worn sunscreen or makeup)
Moisturise	Hydrating toner
SPF50 (EVERY 2 HOURS)	Chemical exfoliation
	Active/treatments
	Moisturiser

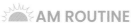 AM ROUTINE

Step 1: Cleanse with a micellar gel wash to remove actives from the night before. It is important that your skin feels hydrated and not tight after this step.
Step 2: Apply a moisturiser without any low-pH actives.
Step 3: SPF50 with skin pH neutral antioxidants is essential to protect against pollutants. Please see 'How to Choose the Best Sunscreen' on page 66 for more guidance. I prefer a mineral sunscreen (zinc oxide) over chemical sunscreen for skin of colour. If you prefer the feel or look of chemical sunscreen, please wear it.

The MOST important thing is to wear any SPF50 cream rather than not wear one at all.

☾ PM ROUTINE

Start your routine at least 2 hours before bed so you have time for actives (the 'hero' ingredients, such as niacinamides, retinol, azelaic acid, etc., which we will get into in depth on page 50) to penetrate, before your face hits the pillow and the product comes off on your sheets.

PM Routine	Product	Purpose
Step 1	Double cleanse	**Removes oily sunscreen and makeup**
Step 2	Hydrating toner	**Hydrates and increases permeability of active ingredients**
Step 3	Chemical exfoliation	**Removes dead skin cells to reveal glowing skin (use 1–2 times a week)**
Step 4	Active/treatments	**anti-ageing/hyperpigmentation/acne etc.**
Step 5	Moisturiser	**Create a healing environment for your skin to repair overnight**

STEP 1: Double cleanse

Start with an oil-based cleanser to remove makeup and any sunscreen.
Follow with a gentle micellar gel wash to remove any remaining products.

Common mistakes:

Using makeup wipes. These tug at your skin unnecessarily and don't remove all the fat-based products on the skin. This can lead to clogged pores.

Over-stripping the skin. The skin should NEVER feel tight or uncomfortable after washing it.

STEP 2: Apply a hydrating, non-alcohol toner

This step will help remove any additional dirt, dust, pollution, bacteria and impurities. It can replenish, soothe and hydrate your skin after cleansing, which is required before exfoliation as it can be a little irritating. This is important for skin of colour, because it can hyperpigment easily when irritated. Make sure you are using a hydrating toner – one that has no denatured alcohol in the ingredient list.

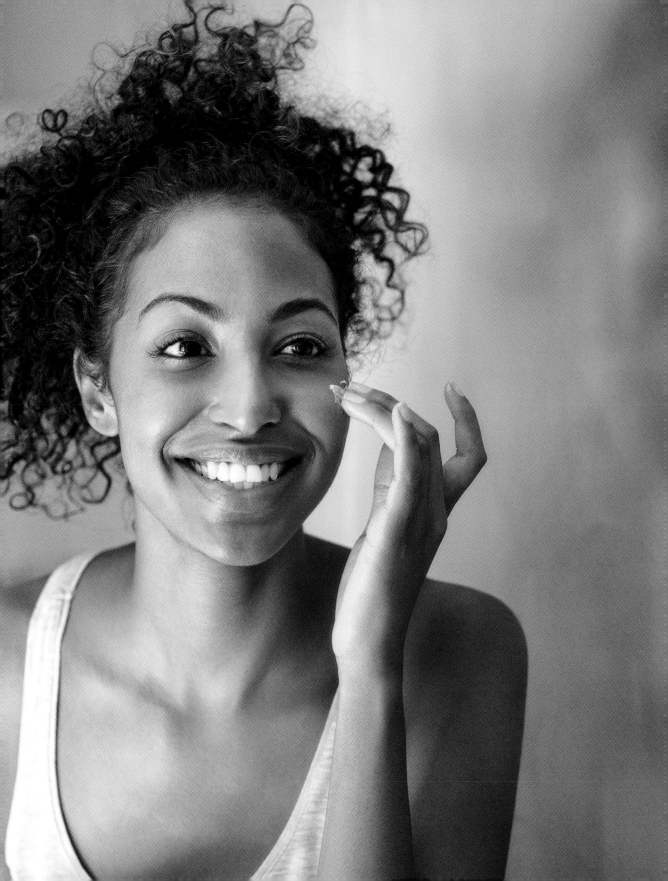

Common mistakes:

Toners used to contain denatured alcohol for its astringent properties to remove excess oil. This actually did more harm than good as often it would increase oiliness of the skin and lead to more breakouts.

Avoid stripping toners that have drying alcohol, fragrance or essential oils.

STEP 3: Exfoliate

Exfoliation is an important step in a skincare routine for several reasons:

- Removes dull skin cells to give a brighter, more even tone.
- Improves permeability of actives, which are skincare ingredients with specific functions.
- Unclogs pores and reduces acne outbreaks.
- Stimulates collagen production.

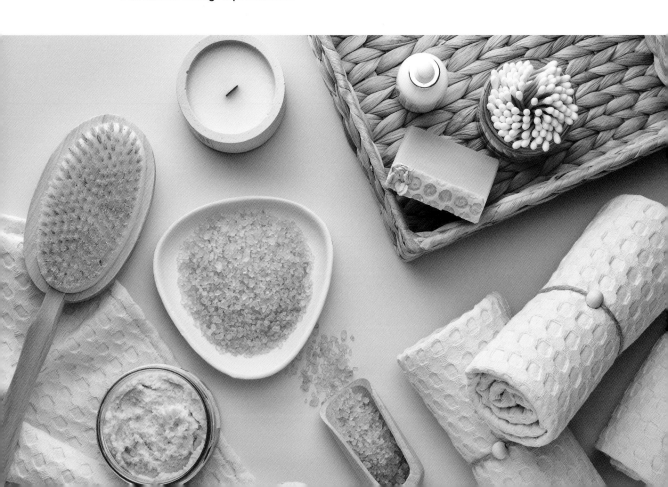

	Example	How it works	How I prefer to use these for skin of colour
Chemical Exfoliation	Mandelic acid Lactic acid Glycolic acid Salicylic acid	**Breaks bonds between dead skin cells so they wash off your skin easily.** **Uniform exfoliation and gentle as it only removes the dead skin cells** **AHAs are hydrating and BHAs unclog pores** **Results take a few weeks to be seen**	For the face, I prefer gentle chemical exfoliation. My favourites are lactic and mandelic acid, as they encourage collagen production and increase cell turnover with minimal irritation.
Physical Exfoliation	Grains Sugar Broken nut shells Sponges Brushes	**Manually removes top layers of skin cells** **Instant brightening of skin but can be too aggressive and cause sensitivity for dry or ageing skin**	I prefer physical exfoliation for the body rather than the face as the epidermis is thicker there.
Enzyme Exfoliations	Papain Bromelain Pumpkin enzyme	**These are proteolytic enzymes that break down the protein keratin into shorter fragments.**	Enzyme exfoliators can sensitise the skin, which is why I am not a fan of them for skin of colour.

Note: I recommend you only exfoliate 1–2 times a week, and do it at night. Take care not to exfoliate too much as it can lead to irritation and flaking. Remember, we want to keep some of the top layer of dead skin cells to protect the skin underneath from environmental factors such as pollution, wind, rain and, of course, the sun.

STEP 4: Active treatments

Why do we apply thinner serums first after cleaning? Serums have a higher percentage of water, which dissolves more active ingredients. They may be able to penetrate the epidermis faster if formulated well. (More advice on how to use actives is on page 50.)

STEP 5: Moisturiser

Moisturiser is all-important – and don't let anyone convince you otherwise. No, your skin's natural sebum production is NOT a substitute for moisturising! There are several reasons why moisturiser is miraculous for your skin.

> **Dull Skin:** If the epidermis is dry, the enzymes (proteases) that break the bonds holding dead skin cells together do not function and this is why dry skin manifests as dull skin. In addition, we need emollients to smooth down the edges of skin cells so we get an even light reflection from the skin.

> **Sensitivity:** Improves erythema (seen as redness or a burgundy shade on skin of colour), flakiness or sensitivity.

> **Ageing Skin:** With age, we lose hyaluronic acid (water magnets) along with fatty acids and ceramides, which act as occlusives, preventing water evaporation from the skin. These are essential for a healthy skin barrier. It is important to maintain this barrier to create a healing environment for your skin. If you use a hyaluronic acid, then you need water molecules to come from your moisturiser, not from deeper in the skin. (Advice on how to choose the best moisturiser for your skin is on page 54.)

Common mistakes:

Correct cleansing, exfoliation, toning all of the expensive active layers – but then you forget the MOST IMPORTANT STEP: moisturiser.

So, now your skincare routine is set, let's find the perfect products for you to use.

How to pick a cleanser

Water is the 'universal' solvent, which means it is able to dissolve more substances than any other liquid. So why isn't it good enough to cleanse our skin?

Two words explain why: surface tension.

An example of surface tension is when I saw a water fountain which was a huge silver ball with water wrapped completely around its shiny surface. How was it possible? Why did the water not fall straight back down? My father, who was my own personal science teacher and was standing beside me at the time, provided the answer: surface tension. It allows water to almost stick together around this globe and not fall straight down. This surface tension is what prevents dirt being cleaned from our skin by water alone.

Surface tension

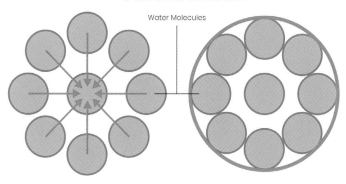

Water molecules being pulled close to each other to mimimise the surface area – meaning the surface tension is higher and harder to penetrate – represented by the sphere

To disrupt the surface tension effect, we need surfactants, which allow water to spread further. They also form dynamic ball-like structures called micelles. That's right, just like micellar water, a term you are probably familiar with from skincare labels.

Micellar structure

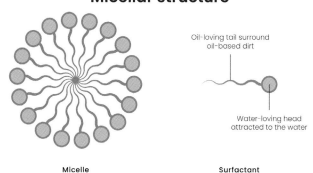

This magical micellar structure is easily washed away by water, which means it's perfectly adapted to cleanse our skin.

Alkyl surfactant such as SLS (sodium lauryl sulphate)

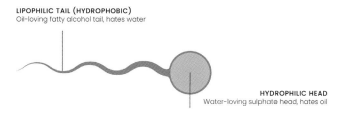

Alkyl surfactants can be quite irritating as they don't discriminate between dirt on the skin and natural skin-barrier oils. This can damage the skin barrier, leading to increased TEWL (Transepidermal water loss), sensitivity and irritation. Any ingredients worn after this will just exacerbate the issue.

Over-washing and over-stripping the skin is the biggest mistake made when cleansing. It is better to use an alkyl ether sulphate, such as sodium laureth sulphate, as a primary surfactant.

What to look for in a cleanser

	Oily and acne skin	Combination skin	Dry skin	Melasma-prone skin	Anti-ageing (If using vitamin A)
Key ingredients	Salicylic acid Sebum control (niacinamide) Benzoyl peroxide (5% if wash off)	Humectants Anti-inflammatory Oil cleanser then gentle micellar gel wash	Humectants Anti-inflammatory Very mild wash May only wash at night	Humectants (healing environment) Anti-inflammatory	Humectants Anti-inflammatory
Your answer to double cleansing	Do not use an oil cleanser	Gel wash in AM Double cleanse in PM	Do not double cleanse	Gel wash in AM Double cleanse in PM	If not dry or damaged barrier you can double cleanse in PM

What is an oil cleanser?

It may seem counterintuitive to use oil to clean your skin. That's because the mechanism that oil cleansers use is different to water-soluble cleansers, which rely on surfactants that engulf oily dirt and make it easier to wash away. An oil cleanser is 'lipophilic', which means they are drawn to oil and fats, such as sunscreen or makeup. This melts the fatty grime, and often agitation is needed to remove the fatty impurities.

For my ageing skin, to which I apply layers of sunscreen to prevent melasma from worsening, I cleanse with my oil-based cleanser first, then wash with a gentle micellar gel wash to remove the oil and any water-based dirt. This leaves my skin feeling hydrated and supple. If I double cleanse with a water-soluble cleanser, my skin feels tight and over-stripped. This is not an optimal 'healing' environment for my skin.

The number one mistake with cleansing is to *over-cleanse* and *over-strip* the skin. This leads to skin sensitivity and a tight and dry skin barrier.

Dr V's Oil Cleanser Recommendations:

- DHC Oil Cleanser (££)
- Paula's Choice Perfect Cleansing Oil (££)
- Face Theory Deeply Nourishing Jojoba Cleansing Oil (£)

How to pick a toner

'Is a toner really necessary?'
'What's the purpose of this step, am I looking to make my skin squeaky clean?'

Originally, toners containing denatured alcohol were used to reduce the 'oil slick' on the skin and minimise pores. They gave a 'squeaky' clean feel to the skin. I will say this now to set the record straight: squeaking is not a sound your skin should be making!

When I was 15 years old, I used a toner for the first time and remember feeling so satisfied removing the dirt from my skin, seeing it on the white pad and hearing that squeak! I thought I was 'doing skincare' perfectly. This was around the same time that I thought I needed to brush my hair 100 times before bed, only to realise my brush had pulled out a fistful of hair! (These are the only two teenage confessions I am willing to share with you all, as I am pretty sure my mum will be reading this book!)

Now we realise that removing oil like this often leads to more sebum production, and over-stripping the skin leads to more sensitivity. Alcohol in toners and other skincare products is used to make a product feel 'lightweight'. However, as it evaporates from the skin, it can lead to dryness, especially if your skin is already dry, sensitive or has a damaged skin barrier.

Instead, what we aim to achieve with modern toners is to:

- Hydrate the skin after cleansing with humectants and skin-restoring ingredients
- Remove excess makeup or dirt
- Mop up free radicals by using antioxidants
- Minimise any inflammation with skin soothers

For these reasons, I like to use a toner *before* I exfoliate.

Double cleanse -> Tone -> Exfoliate -> Actives-> Moisturise -> Barrier oil (If very dry skin)

What to look for in a toner

Avoid:

Denatured alcohol

Witch hazel (that has been distilled in alcohol)

Menthol

Fragrance

Essential oils

Oily and acne skin:

Sebum control, such as niacinamide

Non-comedogenic ingredients

Dry and combination skin:

Humectants, such as glycerin, hyaluronic acid

Anti-inflammatory, such as panthenol, bisabolol, aloe, centella asiatica

Antioxidants, such as green tea and resveratrol

Skin restorers: ceramides

How to choose a toner

Anti-ageing:
Niacinamide, ceramides, peptides

Sensitive/red or burgundy skin:
Hyaluronic acid, antioxidants

Oily skin:
Salicylic acid, niacinamide

Dr V's Toner Recommendations:

Oily skin:

Paula's Choice Skin Balancing Toner (££)
Face Theory Cera-C Pore Reducing Toner (£)
Q+A Niacinamide Daily Toner (£)

Dry skin/combination skin:

Eucerin DermatoCLEAN Face Cleansing Toner with Hyaluronic Acid (£)
The Body Shop Aloe Calming Toner (£)
COSRX - Centella Water Alcohol-Free Toner (££)
PURITO Centella Unscented Toner (££)

How to exfoliate

'Is this really that important, doesn't our skin shed by itself?'
'What exactly does exfoliating achieve?'
'Can I ruin my skin if I do it wrong?'

Exfoliation takes off the top layer of dead skin, exposing juicy younger skin cells and allowing better penetration of actives, which is why exfoliation is so important in a skincare routine. Skin cells turn over roughly every 30 days, but as we age this slows down. As the rate slows down and there is a buildup of dead skin cells on the surface, these become compact and lead to dull-looking skin. The edges of dead skin cells turn upwards and light is not evenly reflected, contributing to the dull skin.

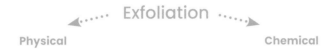

Chemical exfoliation

Chemical exfoliation breaks the bonds holding skin cells together and therefore removes the top layer evenly. With gentle chemical exfoliation, only the top layer of shrivelled, dead skin cells is removed evenly.

This will improve texture, tone and pigmentation of the skin and unclog the pores, which will result in more youthful-looking skin.

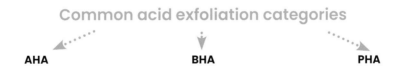

Alpha Hydroxy Acids (AHA):

AHAs are water-soluble and focus on the epidermis. Classical AHAs you will find in exfoliators (with my preferred percentages for skin of colour):

- Glycolic (<5%)
- Lactic (<7%)
- Mandelic (<10%)

Glycolic acid is my least-favourite AHA for skin of colour as it has the smallest molecular weight, and can therefore rapidly penetrate the skin, leading to 'hotspots' and more hyperpigmentation.

Beta Hydroxy Acid (BHA):

BHA is fat-soluble, which means it can penetrate and unclog pores. I recommend:
- Salicylic acid (2%)

Poly Hydroxy Acid (PHA):

PHA works in a similar way to AHA but is a larger molecule, so it doesn't penetrate as deeply or cause as much irritation:

- Gluconolactone or lactobionic acid

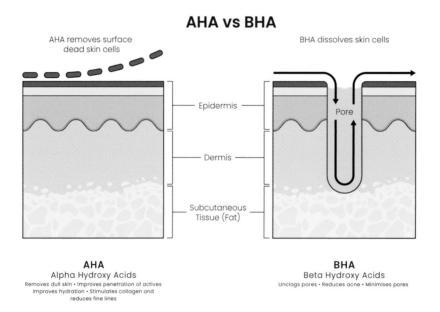

AHA vs BHA

AHA
Alpha Hydroxy Acids
Removes dull skin • Improves penetration of actives
Improves hydration • Stimulates collagen and
reduces fine lines

BHA
Beta Hydroxy Acids
Unclogs pores • Reduces acne • Minimises pores

Physical exfoliation

This is the mechanical removal of skin cells. The problem is, physical exfoliation is often too harsh for skin of colour and relies on using friction to tear off dead skin cells, which is typically done unevenly.

Common physical exfoliants are:

- Scrubs with abrasives
- Face towels
- Whole grains in DIY recipes
- Dry brushes

I once used a well-known face scrub and after several uses I began to notice that my skin felt very sensitive and stung when I applied actives. I could see patches developing on the tops of my cheeks, which had never happened before. Using physical exfoliants had actually resulted in damage to my skin barrier. I stopped using them immediately.

How to choose the best exfoliation method for your skin

Dry and sensitive skin:

Either avoid exfoliation completely or try PHA

Hyperpigmentation, dull or ageing skin:

Mandelic acid and lactic acid

Oily and acne skin:

Salicylic acid

Combination skin:

Mandelic and lactic acid

Dr V's Exfoliating Toner Recommendations:

Oily skin:

Paula's Choice 2% BHA Liquid Exfoliant (££)
Face Theory BHA Exfoliating Serum (£)
Be Minimalist Salicylic Acid 2% (£££)

Dry/combination skin:

The INKEY List PHA Toner (£)
Be Minimalist PHA 3% + Biotic Toner (£££)

Tips for exfoliating safely

If you are concerned about exfoliating, here are a few tips for doing it safely for the best outcomes:

1. Before exfoliation, use a hydrating toner to minimise any irritation and decrease irritation from the double cleanse.
2. After exfoliation, use non-irritating ingredients, like other low-pH ingredients.
3. Avoid using a retinol after exfoliation, as vitamin A increases cell turnover and can further irritate the skin and make it sensitive.
4. Use a moisturiser to help replace hydration of the epidermis.
5. Exfoliate at night to ensure you do not have any UV on the skin after any potential irritation.
6. A common mistake is to over-exfoliate. I recommend maximum twice a week for normal to dry skin.
7. If you have oily skin, it is fine to use your BHA every night.
8. Avoid exfoliation if you have sensitive skin and/or eczema, dermatitis, broken skin barrier, rosacea.
9. Ensure there is no fragrance or drying alcohol in your exfoliator.
10. Ensure SPF50 is worn during the day as skin can be more sensitive in sunlight.

How to use actives

Actives are hero ingredients that we look for in our products – they are heroes because they do a lot of work for our skin. The ones we are familiar with in our teens are salicylic acid or benzoyl peroxide, and as we reach our mid-twenties and lose collagen we start reaching for retinol.

My first experience with actives was for my 'freckle-like' melasma. I learnt about tyrosinase inhibitors quite early on but also made some basic errors. (Read the melasma section on page 156 for my confessions!)

The three main ingredient categories we all need – regardless of skin type – are:
- Antioxidants
- Skin-identical ingredients (those naturally found in the skin, such as ceramides)
- Sunscreen

Even though these are the three main ingredient categories you need, the technology, form of ingredients and feel of the final product will be different per product depending on what the final user requires.
- For dry skin: an oil-based formula or thick emulsion heavy in emollients and occlusives is best.
- For oily skin: use a lighter gel-based formula with no comedogenic ingredients.

This is why the same sunscreen won't agree with everyone.

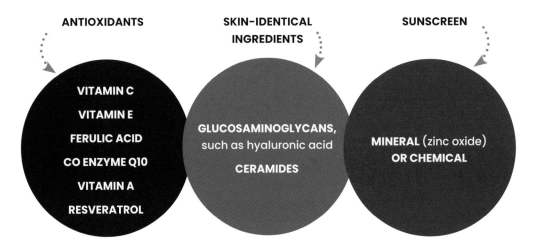

These three categories of actives are the basics, and you can then add in the skin-concern-specific ingredients. For example, for oily, acne-prone skin you may include salicylic acid, benzoyl peroxide, vitamin A, niacinamide and azelaic acid.

Basic treatment ingredient combinations I love

Ageing	vitamin A, hyaluronic acid, peptides, ceramides
Ageing and pigmentation	vitamin A, vitamin C, niacinamide, ceramides, peptides
Acne	salicylic acid, benzoyl peroxide, hyaluronic acid, ceramides, peptides
Dry skin	glycerine, urea, HA, ceramides, peptides, panthenol

Ingredient combinations for specific skin problems

Oily Skin

Control sebum	salicylic acid niacinamide
Increase cell turnover	vitamin A
Mop up excess oil	sulphur clay masks
Hydrate to prevent more sebum	NMF hyaluronic acid

Dry Skin

Humectants	glycerine urea
Occlusives and emollients	paraffinium liquidum petrolatum
Additional barrier oils	squalane hempseed jojoba seed oil

Hyperpigmentation

Melanosome transfer interrupter	niacinamide
Tyrosinase inhibitors	retinoids alpha arbutin kojic dipalmitate vitamin C (such as sodium ascorbyl phosphate and tetrahexyldecyl ascorbate) vitamin E (tocopheryl acetate) green tea extract liquorice extract
Moisturise (humectants)	hyaluronic acid glycerine
Moisturise (occlusives)	paraffinum liquidum petrolatum
SPF50	broad spectrum, such as zinc oxide or tinosorb m

Dull Skin

Exfoliate	mandelic acid lactic acid PHA, such as gluconolactone
Moisturise (humectants)	glycerine sodium hyaluronate lactic acid
Moisturise (occlusives/ emollients)	petrolatum shea butter paraffinum liquidum
Brightening (tyrosinase inhibitors)	vitamin C (sodium ascorbyl/ phosphate and tetrahexyldecyl ascorbate) alpha arbutin potassium azeloyl diglycinate niacinamide

Anti-ageing skin

Exfoliate	mandelic acid lactic acid PHA
Collagen restoration	tetrahexyldecyl ascorbate peptides vitamin A, such as retinaldehyde
Acid mantle restoration (hydrate)	ceramides glycerine urea lactic acid
Antioxidants (prevent further damage)	vitamin E (tocopheryl acetate) vitamin A vitamin C ferulic acid resveratrol green tea

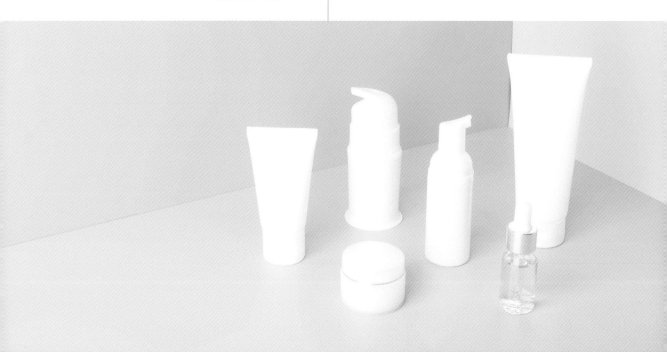

Acne-prone skin

Anti-bacterial	benzoyl peroxide 2–5%
Unclog pores	salicylic acid 2%
Sebum control	niacinamide 2–5%
Antioxidants	azelaic acid up to 10% liquorice root extract
Remove excess oil	clay
Moisturise (light moisturiser)	hyaluronic acid urea

Sensitive/damaged skin barrier

Replace fatty acid	ceramides peptides
Humectants	hyaluronic acid urea glycerine
Occlusives and emollients	paraffinum liquidum petrolatum
Anti-inflammatory	green tea extract aloe panthenol
Additional barrier oil	marula oil squalane rose hip oil

How to choose the best moisturiser

'Does moisturiser actually "do" anything?'
'At night after I apply my serum I feel like my skin is hydrated enough – surely I don't need a moisturiser on top as well?'

Some people think once they have worn their serum their skin feels supple enough, so there's no need to wear a moisturiser on top. This would be a mistake. Serums have a high water content and evaporate quickly, leaving the skin dry with actives on them. This can lead to irritation. Moisturisers are key for a variety of reasons:

Moisturiser improves skin barrier function – cleansing the skin can remove some of our natural skin lipids, leading to some transepidermal water loss due to poor skin-barrier function. This leads to sensitivity and dry skin, which a moisturiser can help to fix.

Moisturiser makes skin glow immediately – dry, shrivelled, dead skin cells stack on top of each other, which means light reflects in different directions so the skin doesn't look smooth. Also, there is less penetration of light.

Moisturiser allows water molecules to separate skin cells so your skin looks plumper, while the emollient ingredients will smooth down the edges of cells so that light reflects evenly. You'll see an immediate improvement as skin is more supple, brighter and glows.

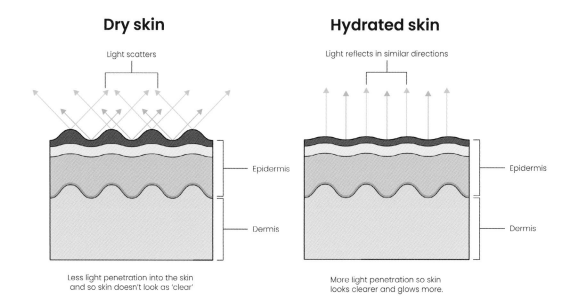

Dry skin

Light scatters

Epidermis

Dermis

Less light penetration into the skin and so skin doesn't look as 'clear'

Hydrated skin

Light reflects in similar directions

Epidermis

Dermis

More light penetration so skin looks clearer and glows more.

Moisturiser improves the appearance of hyperpigmentation – well-moisturised skin means less compaction of dead skin cells. Dead skin cells are stacked together tightly and filled with melanin, the resulting appearance is dull skin and the hyperpigmentation looking even darker.

When you separate these skin cells slightly, hyperpigmentation fades and its appearance improves.

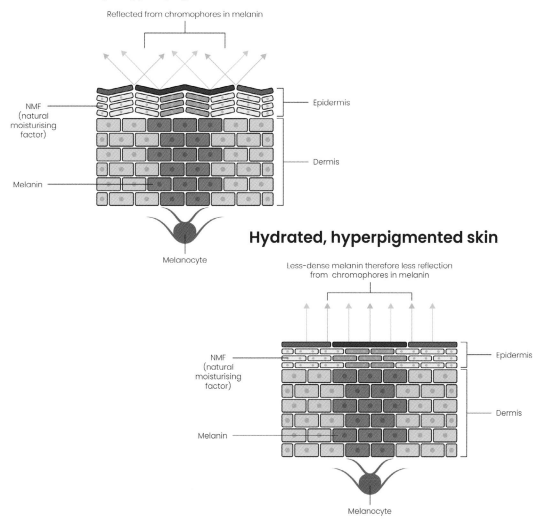

Dry, hyperpigmented skin

Reflected from chromophores in melanin

NMF (natural moisturising factor)

Epidermis

Dermis

Melanin

Melanocyte

Hydrated, hyperpigmented skin

Less-dense melanin therefore less reflection from chromophores in melanin

NMF (natural moisturising factor)

Epidermis

Dermis

Melanin

Melanocyte

Moisturiser helps with anti-ageing – dry skin makes fine lines more prominent; hydrated skin gives a smoother, 'plump' appearance. For enzymes and proteins to function optimally they need to be in a hydrated environment. Constant environmental assault from UV rays or pollution leads to free radicals damaging collagen.

What does optimally hydrated skin look like?

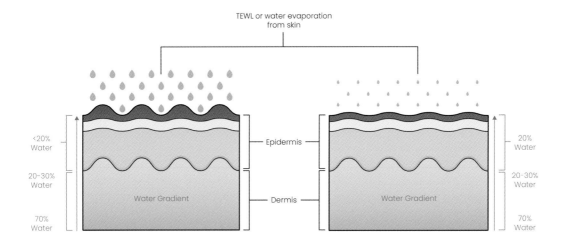

TEWL or water evaporation from skin

	Dry Skin		Hydrated Skin	
<20% Water		Epidermis		20% Water
20-30% Water				20-30% Water
70% Water	Water Gradient	Dermis	Water Gradient	70% Water

Healthy hydrated skin, intact skin barrier

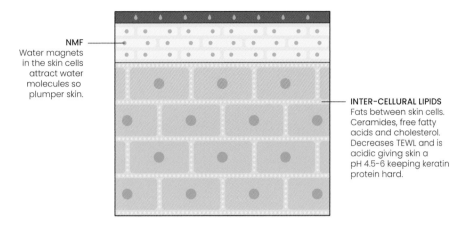

NMF
Water magnets in the skin cells attract water molecules so plumper skin.

INTER-CELLURAL LIPIDS
Fats between skin cells. Ceramides, free fatty acids and cholesterol. Decreases TEWL and is acidic giving skin a pH 4.5-6 keeping keratin protein hard.

What damages your skin barrier?

'Why can't I just add water to my skin to hydrate it above 20% water?'

Increased TEWL leads to dry skin, which damages the skin barrier. This process is triggered by:

• Stress
• Over-stripping the skin (over-cleansing or using alcohol toners)
• Rapid temperature changes
• Dry environment

The reason you can't hydrate your skin with water alone is that it evaporates FAST ...

You need the below to hydrate your skin:

• Occlusives – such as petrolatum
• Humectants – such as glycerine
• Emollients – such as shea butter

'If we need water-loving humectants and oil-loving occlusives and emollients in our moisturiser – how do they mix?'

We all know oil and water do not mix. This is why we use an incredible set of ingredients called **emulsifiers**. Emulsifiers have a water-loving head and an oil-loving tail so they can be held together in an emulsion without splitting back into the separate phases.

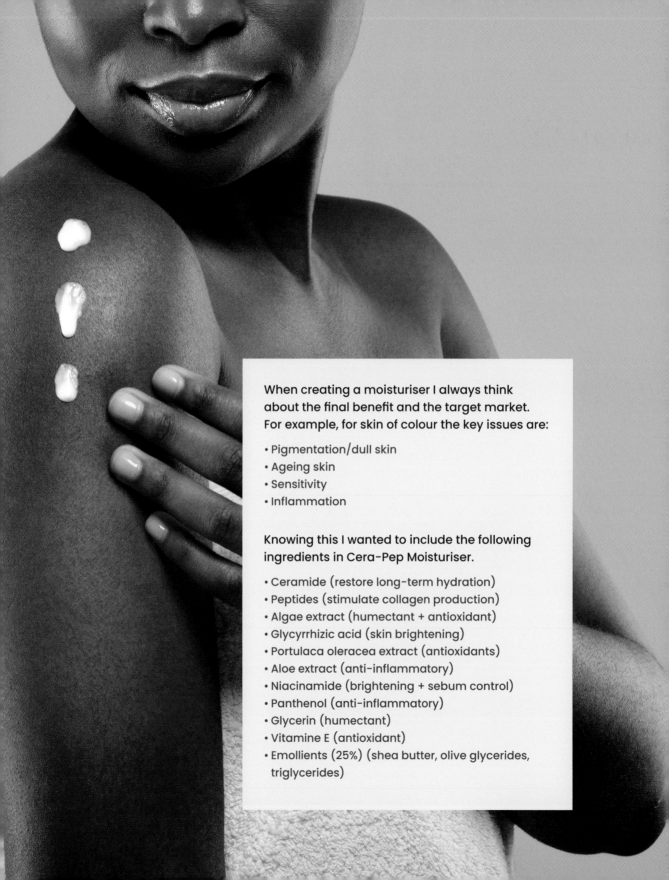

When creating a moisturiser I always think about the final benefit and the target market. For example, for skin of colour the key issues are:

- Pigmentation/dull skin
- Ageing skin
- Sensitivity
- Inflammation

Knowing this I wanted to include the following ingredients in Cera-Pep Moisturiser.

- Ceramide (restore long-term hydration)
- Peptides (stimulate collagen production)
- Algae extract (humectant + antioxidant)
- Glycyrrhizic acid (skin brightening)
- Portulaca oleracea extract (antioxidants)
- Aloe extract (anti-inflammatory)
- Niacinamide (brightening + sebum control)
- Panthenol (anti-inflammatory)
- Glycerin (humectant)
- Vitamine E (antioxidant)
- Emollients (25%) (shea butter, olive glycerides, triglycerides)

Dr V's Formulation Insights

When making Cera-Pep Brightening Moisturiser
I needed to:

- Dissolve ceramides in the oil phase.
- Dissolve niacinamide in the water phase.

Then use an emulsifier with a water-loving end and an oil-loving end to hold the two phases together in an emulsion.

This is also why I run stability tests in the lab, to ensure the oil phase and fat phase don't separate at higher temperatures. And it's why we can have water-soluble and fat-soluble ingredients in a cream.

Creams are just emulsions.

Emulsifier

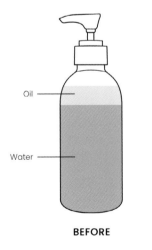

Oil
Water

BEFORE

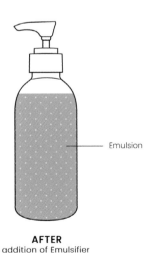

Emulsion

AFTER
addition of Emulsifier

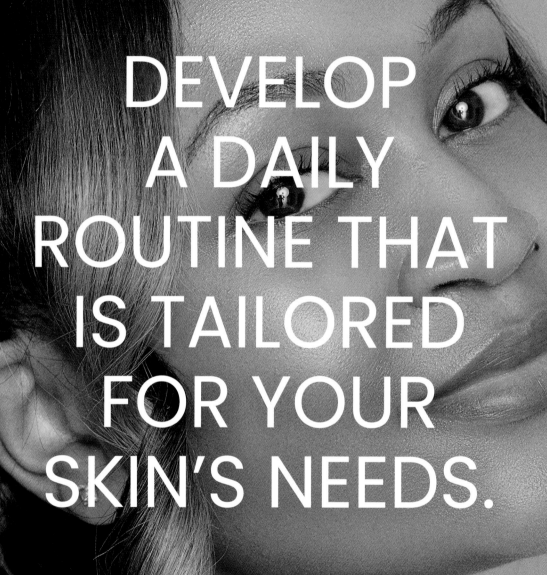

DEVELOP A DAILY ROUTINE THAT IS TAILORED FOR YOUR SKIN'S NEEDS.

Moisturisers are made up of 3 components

Occlusives

Humectants

Emollients

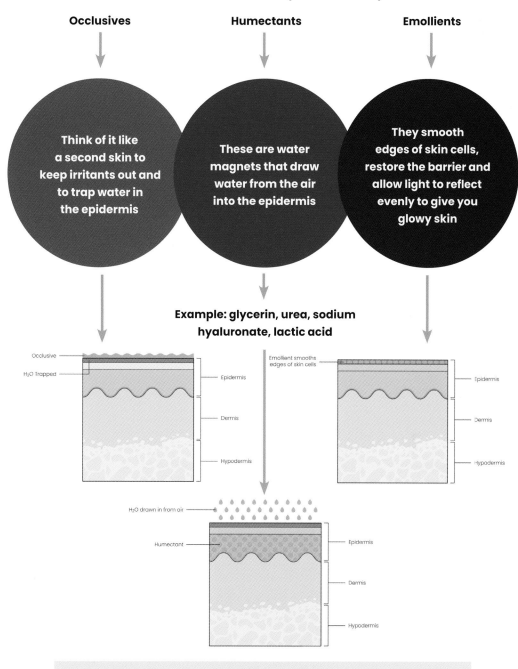

Think of it like a second skin to keep irritants out and to trap water in the epidermis

These are water magnets that draw water from the air into the epidermis

They smooth edges of skin cells, restore the barrier and allow light to reflect evenly to give you glowy skin

Example: glycerin, urea, sodium hyaluronate, lactic acid

Ingredients are often both occlusives AND emollients, e.g.:

DIMETHICONE, LANOLIN, MINERAL OIL, SHEA BUTTER, PETROLATUM

How do you choose the correct moisturiser?

Skin type	Moisturiser properties/ Ingredients	Consistency
Dry skin	high-percentage occlusives/ emollients	cream consistency
Oily skin	non-comedogenic ingredients, light, low-percentage occlusives	gel consistency
Combination skin	hyaluronic acid, ceramides, peptides	cream consistency

Dr V's Moisturiser Recommendations

Oily acne-prone skin:

- Face Theory SuperGel oil-free Moisturiser (££)
- Cetaphil Pro Dermacontrol (££)

Dry skin:

- Cetraben (£)
- VaniCream Moisturizing cream (£)
- QV cream (£)
- Oilatum cream (£)

Combination skin:

- CeraVe (£)
- Be Minimalist – sepicalm 3% + oat moisturiser (££)
- Paula's Choice – Water Infusing Electrolyte (££)

Anti-ageing cream:

- Drunk Elephant protini (£££)
- Naturium Plant Ceramide Rich Moisture Cream (£)
- Hada Labo – anti-ageing super hydrator (££)

Facial oils

I am a big fan of facial oils, especially as a last skincare step in colder and drier seasons for dehydrated, ageing or dry skin. Although they act to keep the skin hydrated, facial oils are not moisturisers – they have a low water content and are used on top of a moisturiser to prevent water loss via evaporation.

During winter months when my skin feels dry and large pores are more prominent in the morning, it is a warning sign that I have not done a good-enough job of hydrating my skin at night. In these situations I step up to **double hydration,** where I apply my fatty moisturiser followed by either squalane or marula oil, which helps to create a healing environment for my skin. This is one of the most important steps for dewy, glowing skin that feels softer and younger.

Heating and air conditioning both dry the skin as they encourage more TEWL. The right facial oils can act as a second skin, decreasing TEWL and keeping the skin hydrated.

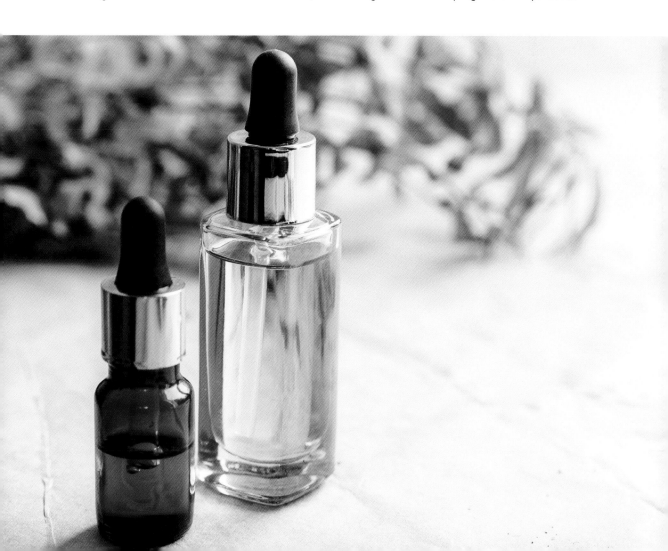

It is important to find the *correct* oil for your skin. The three main categories of oils are:

Fragrant essentials oils – be wary of these as they can increase sensitivity.

Non-fragrant plant oils – my favourites are non-volatile, which do not evaporate at room temperature, because volatility at room temperature can lead to irritation of the skin.

Synthetic oils – can also be good as you can get the benefits you require without the irritation.

Best facial oils

Name	Properties
Borage seed oil	contains gamma linolenic acid, which is moisturising – good for dry skin
Apricot kernels oil	includes emollients and is antioxidant
Argon oil	contains lipids and fatty acids, such as linoleic, vitamin E – is antioxidant
Evening primrose oil	great emollient
Almond oil	contains triglycerides and fatty acids (including oleic, linoleic and myristic)
Jojoba oil	fatty acids – avoid if acne-prone
Grapeseed oil	antioxidant, thinner and easier to absorb as low saturation
Squalane	non-comedogenic, lightweight feel
Rosehip oil	antioxidants and fatty acids

Other less well-known facial oils that I like are:

- Marula oil
- Carrot oil
- Helianthus oil (sunflower seed oil)
- Hemp seed oil (omega 3 and 6 fatty acids)
- Vitamin E
- Lupine oil
- Macadamia nut or peanut oil

Dr V's Facial Oil Recommendations:

The Ordinary: Squalane, Rose Hip Oil (£)
Naturium: Squalane, Marula Oil (£)

Oils to avoid

Fragrant oils and essential oils can be sensitising, unfortunately, when over a long period the skin becomes irritated and skin barrier damage can occur, which leads to sensitivity. Because the effects to the skin are NOT immediate, people continue to use them, worsening the condition. Volatility of fragrant oils on the skin can lead to irritation.

The most common culprits are:

- Citrus oils
- Orange blossom oil
- Grapefruit oil
- Bergamot oil
- Bitter orange oil
- Orange oil
- Lemon or lime oil

Others to look out for and side-step include classic essential oils such as:

- Lavender oil
- Rose oil (not rose hip oil)
- Peppermint oil
- Rosemary oil
- Neroli oil
- Geranium oil
- Eucalyptus oil

My personal skincare routine using facial oils goes like this:

- Double cleanse (take care not to over-wash if skin feels tight or dry)
- Tone (hydrating, non-alcohol toner)
- Exfoliate (avoid if your skin feels dry)
- Treat (use humectants like hyaluronic acid or anti-inflammatory ingredients like green tea extract)
- Moisturise (thick, fatty non-fragrance moisturiser)
- Facial oil (final step at night only)

Dr V's Top Tip:

Only use facial oil as a last step at night. DO NOT wear during the day.

Skincare masks:

The purpose of masking is for occlusion – trapping actives and humectants (water magnets) on the skin to allow better penetration.

This is usually a last step. I prefer either a biodegradable, non-fragranced sheet mask such as an aloe one from The Body Shop or a cream mask from Naturium.

Take care NOT to mask on top of irritants – such as retinol, low-pH acids or fragranced cosmetics.

How to choose the best sunscreen

'What is mineral and what is chemical sunscreen? Are they really that different from each other?'
'How do I choose the correct sunscreen for my needs?'
'When do you apply sunscreen, and can you use it instead of moisturiser?'

Ultraviolet light is a type of radiation that is part of the electromagnetic spectrum. It is emitted by the sun and travels millions of miles to reach Earth – so it's pretty powerful and should be treated with great care. Ultraviolet rays of light (UV rays) can have profound effects on your skin, from increasing hyperpigmentation to accelerating ageing, which is why any skincare routine that doesn't prevent them is severely lacking!

Sunscreen is important all day, every day, but it can be difficult to remember to reapply it when we have such busy lives. Whenever I would go to an outdoor party with a full face of makeup I was terrified of having to re-apply my sunscreen and ruining my makeup, or not re-applying and seeing my melasma darken the next morning. Once, I was at my brother's wedding in Malta in a beautiful location on the roof of a historic fort. With the sun beating down on us, I was forced to make the tough call of re-applying my sunscreen over my makeup. The only two items I was able to bring in my tiny purse were travel sunscreen and eyelash glue (nothing worse than sweat making one eyelash unstick!).

Do you re-apply sunscreen over makeup daily?

Yes (1301 responses)   **No** (6090 responses)

18%   **83%**

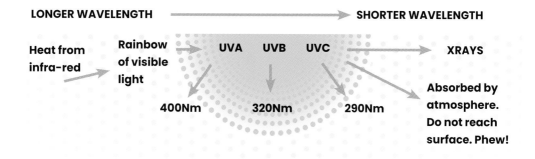

LONGER WAVELENGTH → SHORTER WAVELENGTH

Heat from infra-red

Rainbow of visible light

UVA   UVB   UVC

XRAYS

400Nm   320Nm   290Nm

Absorbed by atmosphere. Do not reach surface. Phew!

UVA

Leads to premature ageing

Various ratings to check for UVA protection:

Boots star rating in UK
UVA logo in Europe
  (symbol of UVA in a circle)
Pa plus rating mostly used in Asia
'Broad spectrum' claim mostly
  used in US

UVB

Leads to burning

SPF rating relates to protecting against UVB rays

UVB rays can damage DNA in skin leading to most skin cancers

SPF stands for Sun Protection Factor and it assesses how many times longer you can stay in the sun before you will be burnt. Although skin of colour is said to have an SPF15, I would never recommend an SPF15 sunscreen, so please do not rely on your melanin for UVB protection. If you do, you are likely to experience premature ageing and hyperpigmentation.

> SPF is mostly a measure of UVB rays.

So, for example, if you normally burn after 5 minutes and you wear SPF50 you are likely to be protected from UVB for 250 minutes. That's assuming there is no sweating, no swimming and no sunscreen shifting.

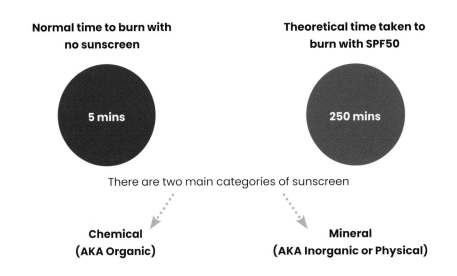

Normal time to burn with no sunscreen

5 mins

Theoretical time taken to burn with SPF50

250 mins

There are two main categories of sunscreen

**Chemical
(AKA Organic)**

**Mineral
(AKA Inorganic or Physical)**

	CHEMICAL	MINERAL
BROAD SPECTRUM/ Stronger UVA performance	Tinosorbs Uvinul A Plus Avobenzone Ecamsule	Zinc oxide Titanium dioxide (for the same particle size, the UVA protection peak for titanium dioxide tends to be slightly lower than that of zinc oxide but it depends on the exact grade used). UV absorbance curves for zinc oxide and titanium dioxide greatly depend on the particle size and shape.
Stronger UVB Performance	Oxybenzone Octinoxate Homosalate Octocrylene	

The ideal sunscreen is broad spectrum, protecting you from UVA and UVB rays.

Your options are:

- Use zinc oxide at a high percentage in a well-considered formulation to optimise the UVB performance.
- Use a combination of UVA and UVB filters formulated together to provide broad spectrum coverage.

Are the mechanism of actions different for mineral vs chemical sunscreen?

Mineral sunscreen pros and cons:

(+) **Mineral –** reflects 5–10% more UV rays than traditional chemical filters. Tinosorb M and Tinosorb A2B are exceptions as they are particulate chemical filters that can also partially scatter UV rays.

(+) **Zinc oxide –** is known to have anti-inflammatory properties.

(+) **Zinc oxide –** is antimicrobial so is a good option for acne.

(+) **Nano zinc oxide –** dispersed evenly in a sunscreen emulsion can be formulated without a white cast. Nano zinc oxide can penetrate the dead top layer of skin called the stratum corneum. If you remember from the skin structure section, blood vessels live in the dermis and nano zinc doesn't make it this far. This means it doesn't enter the bloodstream. Avoid using on broken skin.

(−) If not formulated well or if particle size is too large you are likely to see a 'white cast'.

(−) If not formulated well it's difficult to reach high SPF with zinc oxide alone.

(−) They tend to be more expensive.

(−) They are often not found in chemists.

Chemical sunscreen pros and cons:

(+) These can be much easier to formulate avoiding the 'white cast'.

(+) Newer broad-spectrum UV filters include:
Tinosorb S – Broad spectrum and doesn't penetrate the skin
Tinosorb M – Broad spectrum and can also scatter some UV rays like mineral sunscreens

(+) Tends to be cheaper than mineral sunscreen.

(−) Some chemical filters can change structure when it absorbs UV energy. These changed structures can be irritating to sensitive skin.

(−) Different chemical filters are allowed in different regions across the world. For example, Tinosorb S and Tinosorb M are not currently allowed in sunscreens in the USA.

(−) There is some suggestion that chemical sunscreens can penetrate into the bloodstream and enter breast milk and urine. However, it is worth noting that the amounts are small and may have no adverse effect in our body. We are still waiting for more data on this.

There are pros and cons with both. The MOST important things to remember are:

Do YOU like your sunscreen?
Will YOU wear it 2–3 times a day?
Is it SPF50? (which is essential for melasma and anti-ageing)

I get asked this question a lot:

'What do you prefer for your own skin, Dr V?'

I suffer with melasma and ageing skin that sometimes feels sensitive with the actives that I use at night. This is why I prefer to use zinc oxide SPF50 during the day as I find it soothing and my melasma is under control with it.

If you switched from chemical to mineral sunscreen while using Tyrosinase Inhibitors, did your melasma improve?

YES (632 responses) **NO** (804 responses)

44% **56%**

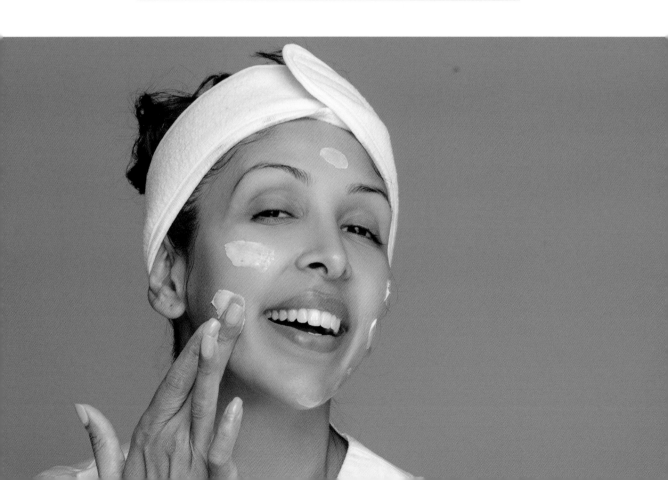

Ingredients I don't like in sunscreens:

- Ascorbic acid – (unstabilised vitamin C) low pH means increased irritation in UV
- Vitamin A – use at night
- Acids – exfoliation increases irritation (don't then go into the sun)
- Ethanol – can dry the skin
- Fragrance – can sensitise the skin
- Essential oils – can sensitise the skin

Ingredients I love in sunscreens:

- Tocopheryl acetate (gentle antioxidant)
- Green tea extract (gentle antioxidant)
- Aloe (gentle antioxidant)
- Centella Asiatica (anti-inflammatory ingredients)
- Arnica (anti-inflammatory ingredients)
- Niacinamide (anti-inflammatory ingredients)

Remember:

- Both mineral and chemical sunscreen must be re-applied to maintain a continuous film of UV protection.

- Both mineral and chemical sunscreen ideally need to dry before you go outside to form an even UV coat of protection.

- Sunscreen rubs off the face just by touching it, using your phone or sweating.

- We often do not use enough sunscreen. The SPF rating is dependent on you wearing $2mg/cm^2$ of skin. In practical terms this is about half a teaspoon. Studies have shown that consumers use $0.5–1.5mg/cm^2$ on average. Make sure you apply sunscreen properly and evenly – apply ½ teaspoon of sunscreen to the back of your hand, then dot it around the face. Rub evenly using the fingertips. The mistake people make is they put it onto the palm of their hand, then rub their hands together, wasting the product and not giving the skin the appropriate coverage needed.

- Sunscreen should be kept cool – for example, pop the container under a towel when on a beach on a hot summer's day.

I prefer MINERAL (zinc oxide) SPF50 to chemical sunscreen for skin of colour, for the following reasons:

1. Zinc oxide has anti-inflammatory properties, which is important for melasma, red marks from acne (PIE) or any form of dermatitis including eczema.
2. Zinc oxide does not enter the bloodstream. Chemical sunscreen (except Tinosorb S) may enter the bloodstream, urine and breast milk. We don't yet know what the effects of this are, if any.
3. Zinc oxide is broad spectrum (as are most chemical sunscreens).
4. It enables 5–10% more reflection of UV rays compared to chemical sunscreen (except Tinosorb M).
5. Nano-zinc oxide, as opposed to non-nano zinc oxide, may be more aesthetically pleasing for skin of colour as it is easier to formulate without a white cast (the white film left behind by sunscreen) and doesn't enter the bloodstream. I have attempted to formulate with both.
6. Zinc-oxide is antimicrobial, which improves my hormonal acne.

This is my personal preference and I want to reiterate – if you like chemical over mineral, please use it. The MOST important thing is that you wear an SPF50 every day.

Behind the scenes: What tests are required to formulate a sunscreen and how long does it take?

Being a cosmetic formulator myself I want to explain why developing a sunscreen is far more challenging than creating most other cosmetic creams. The journey I took to create InZincable™ SPF50 involved rigorous testing of the formulation. We had six rounds of testing in total: from 28 days' testing to see if any reactions occurred on skin, testing the stability of the formula and its compatibility with other common cosmetics ingredients, to patch testing, testing on humans and testing in the lab. All in all, the whole process took about two years.

KEEP YOU AND YOUR SKIN BEAUTIFUL

WEAR AN SPF50

Dr V's Formulation Insights

SPF testing takes longer and the process is more rigorous than for other cosmetic creams.

Usually I can go from idea to formulation to testing to manufacture within 8 months, however, InZincable SPF50 took me almost two years in total from idea to formulating to testing.

If you want to make any claims about a product's effectiveness, you also have to conduct a clinical study.

My aim with InZincable, for example, was to create a mineral zinc sunscreen specifically to prevent and treat hyperpigmentation for skin of colour. This meant it needed sunscreen properties, including:

- Invisible, i.e. no white cast.
- No drying alcohol or fragrance – which is better for sensitive skin.
- UV-stable tyrosinase inhibitors.

I created and Trade Marked a plant stem cell – vitamin complex called 'MelaShield™' – to treat hyperpigmentation for skin of colour and added this to InZincable.

You also need to prove what you created actually works. Usually this is done by engaging a third independent party to conduct a trial on 50+ candidates. The packaging is anonymous for a truly impartial conclusion.

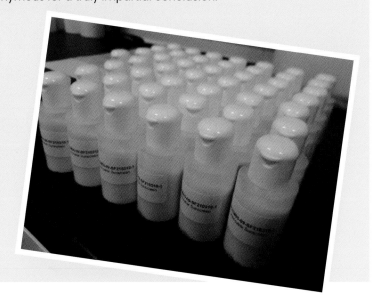

Perfect pores

'My skin looks like an orange peel! How can I minimise these pores?'

This is a question that I may or may not have asked myself while facing the mirror first thing in the morning! Pores are the openings of the hair follicle to the skin. Each follicle has a gland that produces sebum. This sebum then travels up the walls of the pore to create a protective layer from bacteria and environmental stresses such as pollution.

Pores will look enlarged for a few reasons, including:

Genetic – this is the main determining factor.

Over-production of sebum – this tends to get worse during puberty or the week before your period. Over-cleansing or not wearing moisturiser can stimulate further sebum production.

Decreased skin elasticity around the pore opening – this means skin is more rigid and doesn't decrease quickly. This happens with age.

Increased hair follicle volume – when oil, dirt or makeup clog the pores, the pores stretch and look bigger.

Degradation of collagen and elastin.

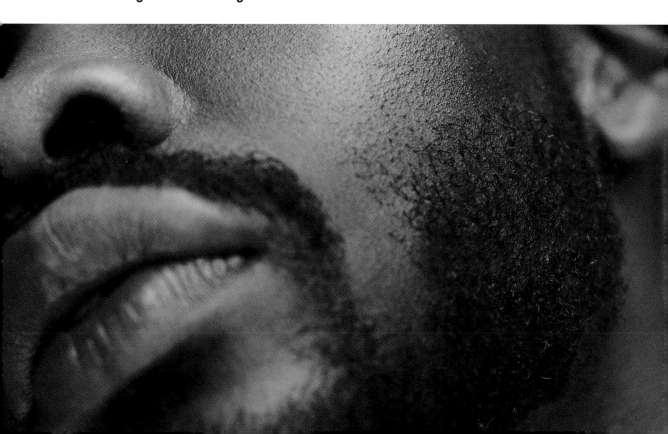

> Reducing the size of pores is important because it will keep skin supple and pores unclogged, reduce over-production of sebum and avoid the degradation of collagen and elastin.

There are a few ways in which you can minimise your pores, depending on your skin type.

If you have oily skin:

- Use a 2% salicylic acid wash or leave-on exfoliant.
- Use niacinamide to control sebum production.
- Use more water-based products and avoid extra oil seeping into pores, opening them up.

If you have ageing, dry skin (like me in the morning!):

- Use a micellar gel wash to clean away dirt and oil and minimise pores.
- Hydrate using a toner and fatty moisturiser containing humectants such as hyaluronic acid.
- SPF50 is essential as sun damage breaks down collagen.

If you have combination skin, follow this routine in the morning:

- Use a micellar gel wash to clean away dirt and oil and minimise pores.
- Use niacinamide on the oily T-zone (forehead, nose and chin).
- Apply moisturiser (gel version for oily T- zone and a fatty emollient for cheeks).

Then follow this routine in the evening:

- Use a micellar gel wash to clean away dirt and oil and minimise pores.
- Hydrate using a toner.
- Apply an antioxidant serum such as vitamins A, C and E.
- Finish with a moisturiser.

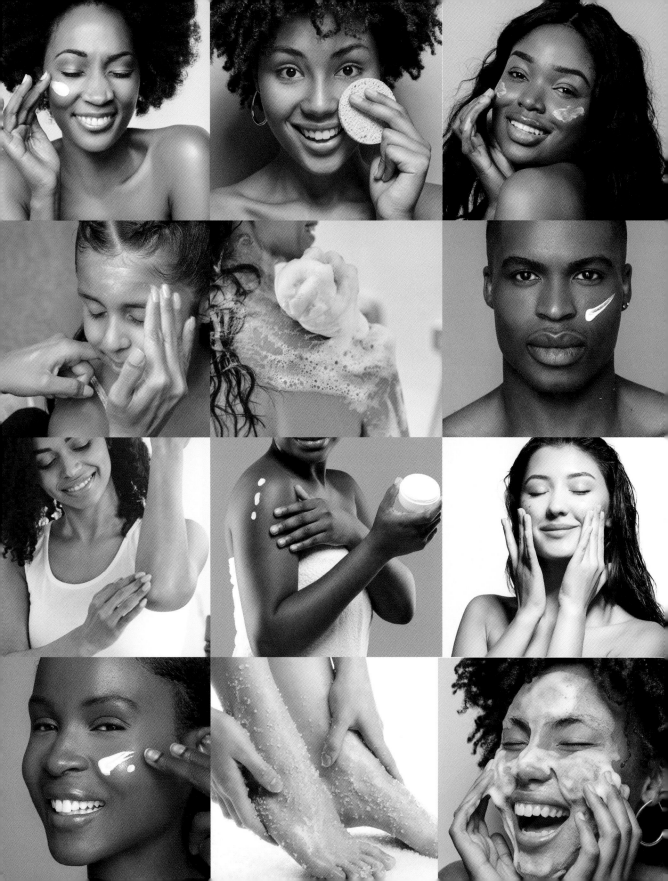

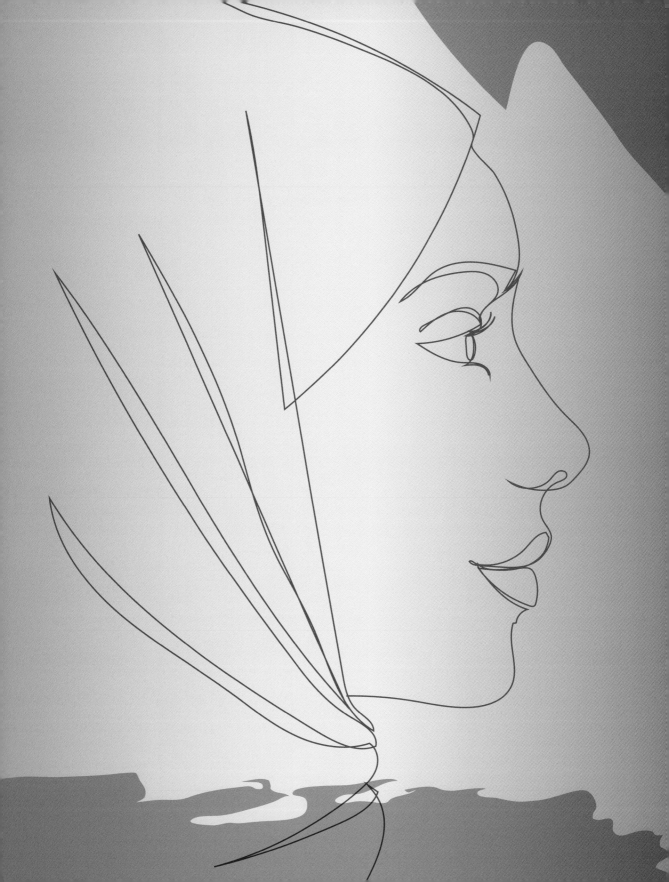

3

INGREDIENTS

Here comes the exciting bit! This is when you will learn how to read the ingredients list on your skincare packaging and decipher when ingredients don't match up to the marketing claims.

I feel this might be the section that the luxury cosmetic cream brands will like the least from this whole book, but this wouldn't be a true Skin Revolution without empowering you – the reader and consumer – to make the best decisions for your skin.

When I began my skincare journey, I didn't know exactly how my skin worked or what it needed, so I trusted the labels on skincare products completely. Having made it my mission to gain precisely this knowledge, I now have a YouTube channel through which I can share this information with my global skin-of-colour family so that they too can have the best skin of their life by understanding the products they are using. After you have read this section you will be able to decode at least half of the ingredients lists in your skincare and you can show off your new skills to your family and friends – and never waste money on the wrong skincare ever again!

Vitamins

We don't just consume vitamins through eating food, they can also be applied topically to protect and improve the structure and function of skin and hair. The correct vitamin applied for a specific problem can have astounding results – for example, vitamin A can improve sagging skin or vitamin C can help reduce pigmentation. It is important to identify the issue and use the correct corresponding vitamin.

Vitamins used in skincare may be derived naturally, however, it is often cheaper to process them synthetically. In addition, vegan cosmetics that are synthetically produced tend to be preferred as natural sources of vitamins A, D, E, K and B12, often come from fish oils, beef liver and egg yolks.

MYTH: Natural is best in skincare

TRUTH: Evidence-based efficacy at a viable price is best in skincare

As a cosmetic formulator, I like to divide vitamins into whether they dissolve in fat or in water. This is important because the skin is waxy (fatty layer), so fat-soluble actives will penetrate more effectively than water-soluble ones. This is why vitamin A should be the first active used on clean skin when layering.

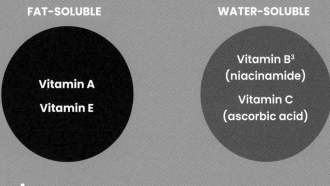

FAT-SOLUBLE

Vitamin A
Vitamin E

WATER-SOLUBLE

Vitamin B³ (niacinamide)

Vitamin C (ascorbic acid)

Vitamin A

'The vitamin A family is royalty in the anti-ageing world'

When we age, we experience more hyperpigmentation, our skin becomes laxer (less firm) and we get more wrinkles. You will likely already know what ageing skin looks and feels like, but what might be new to you is how vitamin A can help with this. To understand how, it is worth digging into the ageing process beyond what we can see on the surface.

What is going on beneath the surface of ageing skin?

- Fibroblasts (collagen-producing cells) produce less collagen.
- UVA rays also induce collagen breakdown (which is why we recommend using a broad-spectrum SPF50).
- More non-functional elastin leads to less 'bouncy skin'.
- An over-production of melanin results in hyperpigmentation and melasma.
- Chronic low-grade inflammation takes place with age.

Here is where vitamin A can help you fight ageing:

- It stimulates collagen production in the dermis.
- It stimulates epidermal skin cells to multiply and assist skin turnover, so there is less time for melanosomes (parcels of melanin manufactured in the melanocyte) to pass into surrounding keratinocytes. This means less hyperpigmentation.

VITAMIN A PATHWAY IN SKINCARE

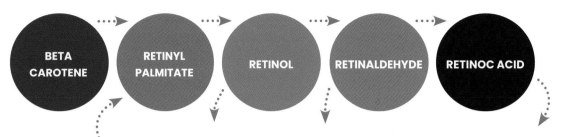

| BETA CAROTENE | RETINYL PALMITATE | RETINOL | RETINALDEHYDE | RETINOC ACID |

WEAKEST VITAMIN A, BUT SAFEST, LEAST IRRITATING.

I recommend this for every night use.

CAN BE IRRITATING/DRYING AND INCREASE SENSITIVITY.

I recommend max 0.5% retinol to minimise irritation for skin of colour.

MY FAVOURITE VITAMIN A FOR SKIN OF COLOUR

Very little irritation.

More effective than retinol.

I love formulating with it for skin of colour.

This ingredient is very expensive though.

MORE POWERFUL AND MOST IRRITATING

Usually need a prescription.

Classic mistakes made with vitamin A

If you used 0.5% retinol or less did you get irritation?

Yes (423 responses)   **No** (1099 responses)

| 28% | 72% |

If you used 1% retinol did you get any redness, irritation, flaking or sensitivity after 1 month use?

Yes (491 responses)   **No** (693 responses)

| 41% | 59% |

There are a few key 'rules' to using vitamin A effectively and without any side-effects:

- Vitamin A is unstable and sensitive to air and light, so robust, airtight packaging is essential to ensure your vitamin A is effective. This is why as a formulator, looking at packaging is just as important as the formulation. I would opt to use an airless, opaque pump when manufacturing an antioxidant serum.
- Apply retinol only at night as it can cause sensitivity. Less irritating vitamin A is fine to wear during the day.
- Make sure you become accustomed to it before you introduce it as part of your regular skincare routine. It is advisable to start applying it on two or three nights a week, then slowly increase application after one month.
- You must wear SPF50 during the day, especially for skin of colour. UV radiation, swimming and sweating all disturb the SPF50 film on the skin. In addition the SPF rating is only effective for 2 hours.
- Do not use vitamin A if you are pregnant or breastfeeding.

What not to combine retinol with:

Another retinol – it is unnecessary and can cause irritation.
AHA – this strips the skin, then when you add vitamin A it is very irritating to the skin.
Benzoyl peroxide – both ingredients individually are irritating. Use separately.
BHA (salicylic acid) – both of these components are drying ingredients. Ensure you moisturise well.

Choose the formulation that is best for your skin

Oily skin – serum or non-comedogenic.
Normal – cream or serum.
Dry – cream with humectants (water magnets, such as glycerine, urea).

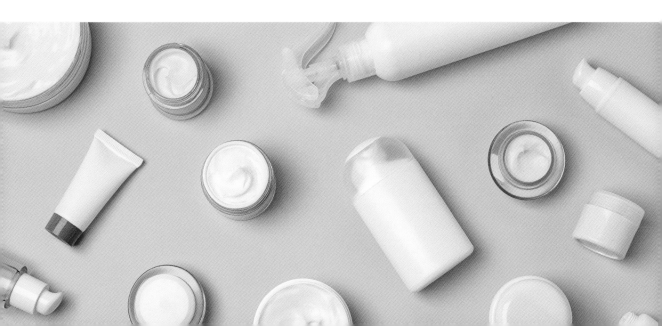

Step by step – how to choose and use vitamin A

How you use vitamin A as part of your skincare routine differs according to the time of day when you are applying it.

🌙 PM ROUTINE

Step 1: Double cleanse (oil wash then micellar gel wash, see page 38) to remove any sunscreen and makeup.

Step 2: Hydrating toner (with humectants, such as urea or glycerine).

Step 3: If you want to use a **daily** vitamin A, **retinyl palmitate** is preferable, and you can apply it directly after toning.

Step 4: Apply any other non-irritating actives, such as niacinamide, green tea extract or hyaluronic acid.

Step 5: Moisturise with a non-fragranced, fatty moisturiser.

> If you want to use **retinol,** apply a fatty moisturiser first to reduce the chances of irritation. ***Don't forget, retinol is an alcohol and you may not be able to tolerate it more than a few nights a week.***

 ### AM ROUTINE

Step 1: Cleanse with a micellar gel wash to remove actives from the night before.

Step 2: Apply a fatty moisturiser.

Step 3: Broad spectrum SPF50 (preferable with zinc oxide as an anti-inflammatory, in case of any sensitivity from vitamin A). Please read the sunscreen section to learn how to choose the best one for your skin (see page 66).

Niacinamide (Vitamin B$_3$)

> *'Niacinamide is everyone's best friend, from acne to pigmentation to sensitivity, and it is also safe to use during pregnancy.'*

Niacinamide is a water-soluble vitamin with many skin-restoring benefits. The pH is 5–7, with a non-irritating profile, which makes it ideal for skin of colour because there is minimal chance of irritation and hyperpigmentation. Niacinamide is a versatile and multi-functional vitamin that is beneficial for your skin in myriad ways and for numerous issues.

> ## Key benefits:
>
> - Decreases lines
> - Decreases hyperpigmentation
> - Decreases erythema (redness or flushed appearance) of the skin
> - Increases elasticity

What can you use niacinamide for?

For hyperpigmentation

- Inhibits melanin transfer from melanocytes to the surrounding skin cells (keratinocytes).
- Good for melasma, post-inflammatory hyperpigmentation, dark circles.

For anti-ageing

- Keeps the skin barrier functioning.
- Hydration and moisture retention.
- Increases collagen and prevents protein glycation from glucose, which helps elasticity.
- Inhibits free radical formulation, which contributes to collagen damage.

For acne (mild/moderate)

- Anti-inflammatory and anti-microbial properties.
- Decreases sebum production.

Helps to reduce pore size

- Niacinamide controls sebum production, which means the pore is less likely to be clogged with sebum and also bacteria.
- Decreases erythema (redness/ flushed appearance) and smooths skin.

Rosacea

- Increases skin barrier function.
- Decreases dryness and sensitivity.

Eczema (aka atopic dermatitis)

- B3 strengthens the skin barrier and reduces redness.

How to use niacinamide in your routine

Niacinamide is UV stable, meaning it is not altered by exposure to daylight and so can be worn both in the morning and at night.

I recommend double cleansing your face and applying niacinamide serum along with any skin-neutral actives, as niacinamide works best at pH 5–7, followed by a layer of moisturiser.

There is some debate about whether you can use niacinamide and vitamin C (ascorbic acid) together. I would advise against applying ascorbic acid (at pH 2.6–3.2) at the same time as niacinamide, as we do not get 100 per cent penetration of actives, so you are wearing two actives that work optimally at different pH levels.

I would suggest that you layer any of the following vitamin C derivatives with niacinamide, because the pH levels are similar and so are working optimally together.

- Sodium ascorbyl phosphate.
- Magnesium ascorbyl phosphate.
- 3-0 ethyl ascorbic acid.
- Ascorbyl glucoside.
- Tetrahexyldecyl ascorbate.

As a cosmetic formulator, it is important for me to look at the optimal conditions for each ingredient individually before we combine them in a cream. After much trial and error, I really like formulating sodium ascorbyl phosphate, tetrahexyldecyl ascorbate and niacinamide into one 'cocktail' cream that is effective for hyperpigmentation or anti-ageing.

Recommended percentage of niacinamide:
There are a lot of 10% niacinamide products available, but I would recommend you start off at 2–5%, as this is the percentage most clinical trials have been based on. In this case – more is not always better.

Did you break out with 10% niacinamide?

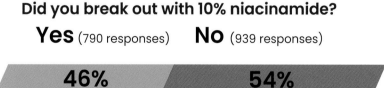

Yes (790 responses)   No (939 responses)

46%   54%

Vitamin C

'Can I wear vitamin C during the day?'
'Can I combine vitamin C with niacinamide?'
'Which are the best vitamin C forms for skin of colour?'

This is one vitamin that we have all definitely heard about – whether it's for fighting common colds or skincare. It has a variety of uses in improving dull skin, hyperpigmentation and texture. In our youth the levels of vitamin C levels in the epidermis and dermis are high, but ageing will deplete these, and that process is exacerbated by environmental assault – such as damaging UV exposure and pollution.

How does vitamin C work with our skin?

- Antioxidants mop up very reactive and damaging free radicals, reducing premature ageing.
- Tyrosinase inhibitors slow the rate of melanin production.
- Boosts collagen levels.
- Vitamin C is a favourite and easily obtainable antioxidant in skin to protect from sunlight, but it is easily depleted.

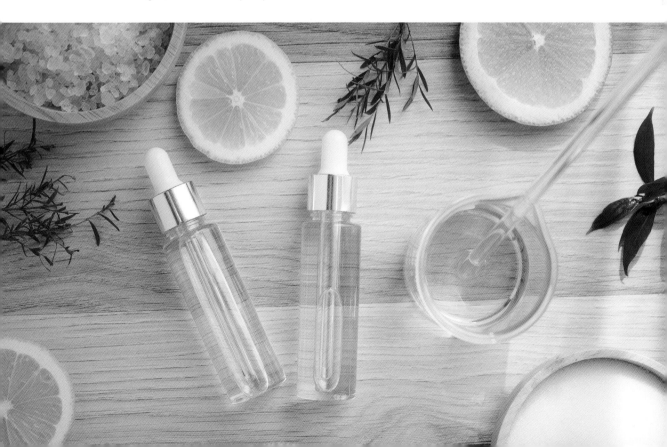

Different forms of vitamin C:

Form of vitamin C	pH	Water-/ fat-soluble	Notes
L-ascorbic acid	pH 2.6–3.2	**Water-soluble**	Very acidic – my least-favourite vitamin C for skin of colour Unstable in light or with oxygen
Sodium ascorbyl phosphate	pH 6	**Water-soluble**	No irritation – converts to L-ascorbic acid stimulating collagen production
Magnesium ascorbyl phosphate	pH 6–7	**Water-soluble**	No irritation – converts to L-ascorbic acid stimulating collagen production
3-0 ethyl ascorbic acid	pH 5–6.5	**Water-soluble**	No irritation – converts to L-ascorbic acid stimulating collagen production
Ascorbyl glucoside	pH 5–8	**Water-soluble**	No irritation – converts to L-ascorbic acid stimulating collagen production
Tetrahexyldecyl ascorbate	**No pH (formulated in oil)**	**Fat-soluble**	Better penetration of the waxy epidermis and reaches the dermis (my favourite form of vitamin C)

L- ascorbic acid – is the most potent type, but it also causes the most irritation and is the most readily broken down with light or oxygen, which then makes it ineffective.

Sodium ascorbyl phosphate, magnesium ascorbyl phosphate, 3-0 ethyl ascorbic acid and ascorbyl glucoside – all convert to L-ascorbic acid in the skin. This means they cause less irritation but they are less effective than L-ascorbic acid. They are also more stable and not as easily broken down.

Tetrahexyldecyl ascorbate – is my favourite form of vitamin C, because the first issue for any skincare ingredient is penetration of our waxy, waterproof skin, and fat-soluble ingredients like this improve penetration. It is also stable and not easily broken down.

Packaging is important for vitamin C because it is very unstable in the presence of light and oxygen. It should be packaged in an airless, opaque pump and used in combination with other antioxidants to stabilise it, such as green tea extract or vitamin E.

The biggest questions with vitamin C are:

How much of the product has broken down before use?

How much actually penetrates the epidermis?

Which forms are best for skin of colour?

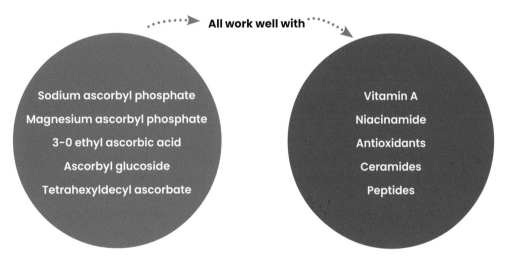

Dr V's Formulation Insights

I tend to formulate with a cocktail of sodium ascorbyl phosphate and tetrahexyldecyl ascorbate together, giving me a stable formula that combines both water and fat-soluble vitamin C.

Good combinations for vitamin C:

All work well with

Sodium ascorbyl phosphate
Magnesium ascorbyl phosphate
3-0 ethyl ascorbic acid
Ascorbyl glucoside
Tetrahexyldecyl ascorbate

Vitamin A
Niacinamide
Antioxidants
Ceramides
Peptides

Which vitamin C can I wear during the day, and which at night?

To minimise chances of irritation, please only wear L-ascorbic acid at night.

During the day you are unlikely to get any sensitivity if you are wearing:

• Sodium ascorbyl phosphate
• Magnesium ascorbyl phosphate
• 3-0 ethyl ascorbic acid
• Ascorbyl glucoside
• Tetrahexyldecyl ascorbate

Best and worst acids for skin of colour

'Acids are scary – I tried a TikTok trend and burnt my skin.'
'I have no idea which acid is safe for my skin.'
'How do I layer acids?'

What is an acid, how is it used on our skin, which ones are safe for skin of colour and at what percentages should we be using them?

Acids in skincare have varying strengths and all have different impacts. Our skin is already slightly acidic, which is why we can use a weak acid in a formulation to improve the penetration of ingredients, but also because stronger acids will exfoliate the skin and acids that are too strong will burn the skin and lead to hyperpigmentation.

I remember when I first heard about using acids in skincare, my instant reaction was 'never will I do that to my face!' This is the natural fear instinct that we have before we understand something and watch others use acids successfully.

The fundamental problem is following people who have no knowledge of skin and who make DIY skincare concoctions with lemon juice and apple cider vinegar with the strapline: 'If it is good enough for you to eat, it is good enough for your face.' My response to this is, 'Your face is NOT a salad!' These acids are far too irritating for skin of colour and can lead to hyperpigmentation.

Salicylic acid (also known as beta hydroxy acid or BHAs)

This is one of my all-time favourite acids for skin of colour!

It is a fat-soluble acid, which means it will penetrate the sebum-filled pores easily and unclog them, which makes it ideal for treating white heads and black heads. It also reduces excess oil in pores, which helps to shrink the appearance of pores.

Its anti-inflammatory properties also help to reduce erythema from breakouts, such as red and burgundy marks from Post-inflammatory Erythema (PIE).

Dr V's salicylic acid recommendations:

The Ordinary Salicylic Acid Mask 2% (££)
Be Minimalist Salicylic Acid 2% (££)
Boots Ingredients Salicylic Acid Serum (£)
Paula's Choice Skin Perfecting 2% BHA Liquid (££)
Naturium BHA Liquid exfoliant 2% (££)
Face Theory BHA Exfoliating Serum S3 (£)

Who is it for?

This is ideal for use on oily and acne-prone skin or enlarged pores (<2% salicylic acid) and to use to exfoliate thickened skin (>5% salicylic acid).

Potential side-effects:

Dry skin and some flaking.

What NOT to combine it with:

Avoid using with other forms of exfoliation. Do not use another product with salicylic acid in your routine with this. You can find salicylic acid in washes, toners, exfoliants, creams and serums.

What to combine it with:

- Humectants, such as glycerine, urea, hyaluronic acid.
- Anti-inflammatories, such as green tea extract, panthenol.
- Others: Niacinamide to minimise pores or improve acne.

Who should avoid it:

Don't use on dry, eczema-prone skin. Alternatively, use it as a spot treatment, but not on the whole area.

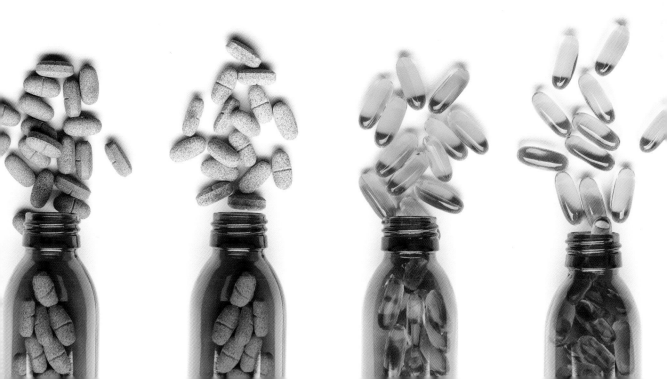

Hyaluronic acid

This is a confusing one because it sounds like an exfoliator but it is actually a humectant (a water magnet that hydrates the skin). Hyaluronic acid plumps up the skin and reduces the appearance of wrinkles. This 'healing' environment improves wound recovery time, too.

One hyaluronic acid molecule attracts and holds almost 1,000 times its weight in water

In a humid environment water molecules come from the atmosphere. In a dry environment, like in a desert, or during winter in the UK, water molecules come from deeper in the epidermis, making your skin feel drier and tighter. You must wear a moisturiser on top and it may help to use a cool-air humidifier at night. It is found in face washes, toners, exfoliators, serums and moisturisers. This is an expensive ingredient, so I prefer to use it in a leave-on product as opposed to a wash-off product.

Who is it for?

Hyaluronic acid is for ageing and dry skin. It also helps with a damaged skin barrier.

Ageing skin is drier and holds fewer water magnets (glucosaminoglycans), which makes it so much harder to hydrate the skin, and this worsens the appearance of wrinkles.

What to combine it with:

• Niacinamide, vitamin C

Glycolic acid (an Alpha-hydroxy acid or AHA)

Glycolic acid is the smallest AHA molecule and flies through the skin quickly. The benefits are that it dissolves sebum, pore plugs and dead skin cells. This can improve the appearance of pigmentation and smooth out wrinkles.

Despite the popularity of glycolic acid, it is my least-favourite AHA for skin of colour as an exfoliant because of its molecular weight. Its ability to fly through the skin makes skin of colour susceptible to 'hot spots', burns or PIH. Most people using glycolic acid will be fine, but my aim has always been how to achieve maximum results with minimal chances of burns.

I would use it at maximum 5% for skin of colour to minimise chances of irritation. In the laboratory, I like to formulate with it as a 'surgical knife' at the cellular level, to help improve penetration of other actives for areas of thicker skin, such as on elbows and knees. However, I prefer other AHAs with a larger molecular weight than glycolic acid for exfoliation purposes, such as mandelic acid and lactic acid.

Potential side-effects:

High-strength glycolic acid can cause irritation, inflammation, scarring, discolouration, stinging, burning, crusting or scabbing.

These side-effects depend on the percentage used and the condition of your skin, e.g. your skin sensitivity – if any other skin conditions are present, the skin is dry, the skin barrier is compromised or what other ingredients are being used in conjunction. This is why I prefer lactic acid or mandelic acid for skin of colour.

What NOT to combine it with:

Any other high-percentage exfoliating acids, denatured alcohol, essential oils or fragrance. You don't want to mix an already irritating ingredient with other known irritants. Avoid mixing it with retinol or ascorbic acid.

What to combine it with:

- Humectants: urea, glycerine
- Anti-inflammatory: green tea, chamomile, panthenol, *Centella Asiatica*
- Ceramides and peptides
- SPF50 during the day is essential due to the skin's increased sensitivity to UV.

Who should avoid it:

Anyone with dry or sensitive skin, where dermatitis is present or there is a damaged skin barrier.

Lactic acid (also an AHA)

Lactic acid is a gentle, exfoliating AHA with a larger molecular weight than glycolic acid. This is why it doesn't penetrate the skin as deeply and is unlikely to lead to burns or 'hot spots'. It improves fine lines, decreases the appearance of hyperpigmentation, and increases cell turnover. This results in younger, plumper skin cells coming to the surface faster and gives you a glowing complexion. Lactic acid is a hydrating acid, which polishes and exfoliates the skin, so I would exfoliate once a week with it to improve penetration of actives. You can use it all year round, and apply at night to maximise its hydrating properties.

What NOT to combine it with:

Physical exfoliation, retinol, ascorbic acid.

What to combine it with:

- Humectants: urea, glycerine.
- Anti-inflammatory: green tea, chamomile, panthenol, *Centella Asiatica*, Ceramides and peptides.
- SPF50 during the day is essential due to skin's increased sensitivity to UV.

Who should avoid it:

Anyone with a damaged skin barrier or dermatitis.

Mandelic acid (also an AHA)

Mandelic acid is a large molecular-weight AHA, and because it is large, it slowly penetrates the dermis and loosens the connections between the skin cells (keratinocytes) called desmosomes. This allows dead skin cells to slough off, to reveal brighter skin. Increased cell turnover will improve hyperpigmentation, acne and fine lines.

Who is it for?

It is suitable for acne, anti-ageing and hyperpigmentation in skin of colour.

Potential side-effects:

These are very rare, but it can sometimes increase sensitivity to UV.

What NOT to combine it with:

Retinol, physical exfoliation (including using it on newly waxed or shaved skin).

What to combine it with:

- Most other actives work well with mandelic.

Azelaic acid

A gentle, exfoliating acid that penetrates the pores and decreases keratin (a protein that makes dead skin cells stick together and unable to leave the hair follicle), therefore preventing plugs from developing and brightening the skin.

> It is an antibacterial that reduces the growth of the most common acne-causing bacteria (Cutibacterium acnes or C. acnes) in your follicles.

Azelaic acid normalises sebum production and is also a tyrosinase inhibitor, and so helps with hyperpigmentation. This is why it works well for brown acne marks (Post-inflammatory Hyperpigmentation, PIH). It has anti-inflammatory and antioxidant properties, too, which helps with Post-inflammatory Erythema (PIE) – the red or burgundy marks from acne and Rosacea.

Azelaic acid has a pH of 4.6 and is one of my favourite acids for skin of colour, triggering very few adverse reactions.

I tend to take it one step further and use a potassium azeloyl diglycinate derivative, because it is easier to formulate with, lower percentages are effective and it is more hydrating and therefore better for skin of colour. I formulate this at the same pH level as skin, which is approximately 5.5. This means even less irritation, plus the moisturising benefits of glycine.

Who is it for?

For acne and marks caused by acne, sensitive skin and pregnancy skincare.

What to combine it with:

- Use an AHA or BHA first to exfoliate the skin and improve penetration of the azelaic acid.

Alcohol in skincare

Why would alcohol be needed in skincare? There are two main reasons why it is used. Short-chain alcohols are used to give a lightweight texture to a formula, and this is particularly common in sunscreens, which are typically heavy if they are poorly formulated. The second reason is that long-chain alcohols are used as emollients.

The two categories of alcohols have completely different properties based on their molecular weight. When formulating for skin of colour, I try to find a way to deliver maximum efficiency with the least irritation, which is why I avoid formulating with short-molecular weight alcohols. On the flipside, I highly recommend long-chain fatty alcohols especially for dry, ageing skin of colour.

	Short-chain alcohol	Long-chain/Fatty alcohol
PURPOSE	Solvent	Emollient
	Lightweight texture to a cosmetic formula	Smooth skin cells
	Improves spreadability	
PROPERTIES	Evaporates quickly	Does not evaporate
	Dehydrates the skin	Traps water in epidermis
	Disturbs skin protective barrier	Solid, white and waxy at room temp
NAMES	Denatured alcohol	Cetyl alcohol
	Ethanol	Cetearyl alcohol
	Propanol	
	Isopropyl alcohol	
COMMONLY SEEN IN	Sunscreens	Conditioners
	Moisturisers	Moisturisers

Collagen

'Are collagen creams and supplements actually anti-ageing?'
'Which is the best form of collagen?'
'When should I start using collagen?'

Collagen is the main structural protein in the dermis and it provides strength to skin. It is found in skin, cartilage, membranes, organs and bones – it's actually the most abundant protein in the body!

What happens to collagen as we age?

I clearly remember being at medical school when my dad said to me, 'Vanita, you are now 21 years of age, this is the peak for your skin, it is downhill after this!' Although this was pure scientific fact, I remember feeling mortified and saying, 'But, Dad, I haven't actually lived my life yet, I have spent it all studying!'

Collagen production decreases by about 1% each year after 21 years of age, which causes the firmness of the skin to decrease. Collagen loss can occur even more rapidly during menopause.

There are two steps we need to consider when thinking about collagen in skincare.

Step 1: The slow rate of collagen breakdown
Step 2: How to stimulate collagen production

What damages collagen?	How to combat this:
UV rays	SPF50
Pollution	Antioxidants topically and diet
High sugar leads to glycation	Avoid a high-sugar diet
Smoking	Stop smoking

More wrinkles and loss of suppleness can also result from glycation, which is when a sugar molecule binds to the elastin and collagen protein.

Supplements vs creams

Intuitively we think if we consume collagen or use it in creams it all goes into restoring our natural collagen and keeping us looking young. This isn't quite the case. Marketing claims with collagen in the ingredients list include the ability to restore collagen in the skin.

*Collagen has a large molecular weight and it **cannot** penetrate the epidermis.*

Collagen behaves like a moisturiser when applied topically – so when it is applied, it does not actually enter your skin in the way you might hope for.
So what are your options for stimulating collagen production in skincare?

Category	Ingredient names
Vitamin A	Retinyl palmitate, retinol or retinaldehyde
Fat-soluble vitamin C	Tetrahexyldecyl ascorbate
Antioxidants	Vitamin E, resveratrol, green tea extract
Skin repairers	Peptides, ceramides, hyaluronic acid
Chemical exfoliation	Lactic acid + mandelic acid is my favourite combination for skin of colour

WHEN I
BEGAN MY
SKINCARE
JOURNEY, I
DIDN'T KNOW
WHAT MY
SKIN NEEDED

Do collagen supplements work?

Taking collagen in supplement form has been shown to:

- Improve skin hydration
- Aid skin elasticity
- Reduce wrinkle depth

The recommended dose is 2.5–8 grams per day for 8 to 12 weeks, after which you will start to notice a difference in your skin, hair and nails. A clinical study of 69 women between 35 and 55 years old who consumed 2.5–5 grams of collagen daily for 8 weeks resulted in an improvement in skin suppleness[1].

After the birth of my two children, I suffered hair loss and decided to take 6–8 grams collagen daily. Although I am not a vegetarian, I do not count how many grams of protein I eat each day (collagen is a protein). In addition to taking the collagen supplements, in my laboratory I made a topical serum for my scalp with vitamins, antioxidants, peptides and anti-inflammatory ingredients to improve my hair growth. I made a hair oil to strengthen the hair shafts and smooth hair cuticles. This meant less breakage. I also used an infra-red cap to stimulate my hair follicles. When I tackle a problem I tend to read every piece of research and figure out how it can be combined. Hair growth does ideally require this dual internal plus external action for maximum benefit – and I'm pleased to report that my plan worked!

Tyrosinase inhibitors

'How do they reduce hyperpigmentation?'
'Which ones do I use and how do I layer them?'

This is a term that everyone who has hyperpigmentation should know. Tyrosinase inhibitors are a category of ingredients that slow the rate of melanin production, which in turn reduces hyperpigmentation. The problem is that not all tyrosinase inhibitors are suitable for skin of colour – some work better together and others should not be worn together.

So, to make this less confusing, I will break it all down for you here. Firstly, you may wonder if treating hyperpigmentation is the same as skin lightening (which aims to depigment the skin). This confusion occurs because tyrosinase inhibitors slow down the rate of melanin production in your skin. However, skin-lightening products can be incredibly damaging to skin and while they may use tyrosinase inhibitors, they do so in different formulations, which might also include toxic bleaching agents such as mercury. Some use unregulated IV glutathione drops, which can damage organs and others contain hydroquinone, which must be supervised by a doctor and should never be purchased over the counter. In my clinic, I have unfortunately seen too many people burn their skin with unregulated skin-lightening creams. Hyperpigmentation treatment only aims to even a person's normal skin tone.

Tyrosinase Enzyme

Tyrosinase is the 1st step in melanin production (pigment in our skin).
This enzyme CONVERTS the tyrosine in our skin into melanin.

HOW TYROSINASE IS STIMULATED

External trigger:

UV radiation
Menopause, the pill
Insect bite
Chemical/heat burns
Trauma
Friction (inner thigh/knees/toes)
Cosmetics irritation, such as lip
  pigmentation

Internal trigger:

Hormonal, such as puberty,
  pregnancy
Hereditary, such as dark circles, aka
  periorbital pigmentation
Acne

From trigger to HYPERPIGMENTATION

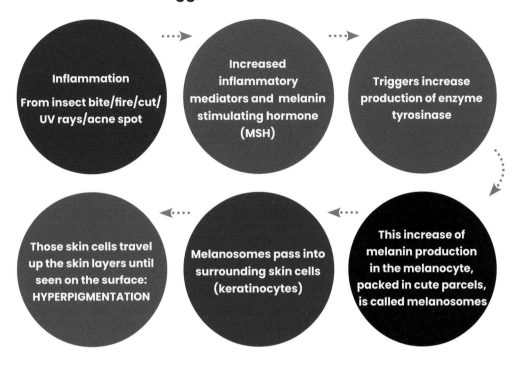

Inflammation

From insect bite/fire/cut/ UV rays/acne spot

Increased inflammatory mediators and melanin stimulating hormone (MSH)

Triggers increase production of enzyme tyrosinase

Those skin cells travel up the skin layers until seen on the surface: HYPERPIGMENTATION

Melanosomes pass into surrounding skin cells (keratinocytes)

This increase of melanin production in the melanocyte, packed in cute parcels, is called melanosomes

Some of my favourite tyrosinase inhibitors for skin of colour:

- Retinoids
- Alpha arbutin
- Kojic acid or kojic dipalmitate
- Vitamin C
- Vitamin E
- Green tea extract
- Liquorice extract

For skin of colour I tend to formulate with all of the above plus niacinamide. Niacinamide interferes with melanosome transfer from melanocyte to keratinocyte, which means less melanin is produced so you see less hyperpigmentation.

Hyperpigmentation is a stubborn condition to treat, especially periorbital pigmentation (dark circles around the eyes). Often one to two of the actives from the list above won't be enough, but I recommend 8-10 Tyrosinase inhibitors for stubborn pigmentation around the eyes.

How tyrosinase inhibitors work

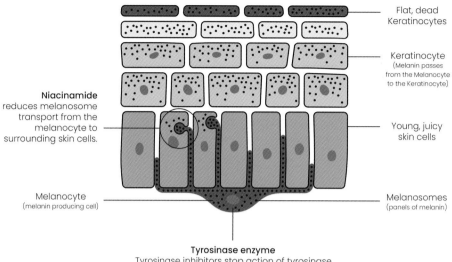

Flat, dead Keratinocytes

Keratinocyte
(Melanin passes from the Melanocyte to the Keratinocyte)

Niacinamide
reduces melanosome transport from the melanocyte to surrounding skin cells.

Young, juicy skin cells

Melanocyte
(melanin producing cell)

Melanosomes
(panels of melanin)

Tyrosinase enzyme
Tyrosinase inhibitors stop action of tyrosinase so it never becomes melanin.

Dr V's Formulation Insights

I instructed a third-party independent clinical trial on our Dr V tyrosinase-inhibiting kits in order to determine the most effective percentages we should be using that work well in combination and cause the least amount of irritation to skin of colour.

With my Lip Hyperpigmentation (Dr V Lip-X), we titrated up (increased) from using three tyrosinase inhibitors in one product and not seeing any results in the clinical trial to using eight tyrosinase inhibitors over a three-product kit and seeing 100% of trial candidates seeing a reduction in their lip pigmentation.

This is a strong indicator that treating hyperpigmentation in skin of colour requires a cocktail approach, as opposed to layering single active ingredients, because this skin condition is very stubborn to treat.

Ingredients to avoid in skincare

On social media I am well known for recommending that you avoid the below in your skincare products:

- fragrance
- drying alcohols
- essential oils

This opinion can lead to much controversy, especially from manufacturers who have products that include these ingredients and from agents who make commission selling their products. I do tend to receive a fair number of angry emails on this subject. I fully understand the perspective of formulators who use fragrance, but I also see the industry changing and responding to these points.

Most people are absolutely fine using fragrance and drying alcohol on the skin and suffer no side-effects or reactions, but for me, the stakes are higher. To date, my YouTube channel has had 30 million views, and if I recommend a product with even a 1% chance of irritation or inflammation, this can mean tens of thousands of my skin-of-colour followers potentially damaging their skin barrier or seeing hyperpigmentation.

I always ask two questions of any product:

Can it cause irritation?
How effective is it?

So here I want to do a deep dive into fragrance, drying alcohols and essential oils.

There are **26 substances listed in Annex III of EU cosmetic regulations that are considered to cause allergies.** Fragrance and essential oils have the most allergic potential; in fact, 1–2% of people are considered to have an allergy to fragrance.

The following known allergens can be manufactured synthetically or derived naturally, so this is NOT a 'natural is better than synthetic' issue, or vice versa.

- Anise alcohol
- Benzyl alcohol
- Benzyl benzoate
- Benzyl cinnamate
- Benzyl salicylate
- Cinnamal
- Cinnamyl alcohol
- Citral
- Citronellol
- Coumarin
- Eugenol
- Farnesol
- Geraniol
- Isoeugenol
- Limonene
- Linalool

The ingredients I see most regularly on cosmetic packaging during my investigations include:

- Cinnamal
- Citral
- Citronellol
- Coumarin
- Geraniol

This can be confusing if you don't know that, for example, 'citral' is a fragrance.

Essential oils tend to include limonene – such as those fragranced with lemon, peppermint, lavender, bergamot or orange. Linalool is found in lavender, lemon, apple, rosewood, pine or apricot oils.

> *As you can see, many of these allergies are to natural ingredients, or those that are included in essential oils, which are widely considered a good thing in skincare.*

In the EU, any leave-on product like a cream must show the allergen in the ingredients list if it is present in amounts of more than 0.001%. For a wash-off product you need to declare it if the percentage is more than 0.01%

This is why body washes and shampoos are so heavily fragranced compared to creams, because you are allowed to formulate with it at a higher percentage without having to disclose it (for example, if it is just less than 0.01%). I also wanted to write out the names of these ingredients so you can check your creams and makeup for them, as often the INCI name used is not simply the word 'parfum'.

Essential oils can be confusing as they can have benefits – for example, anti-inflammatory, anti-bacterial and calming. However, as they contain potential allergens the risk–reward ratio doesn't stack up. I would rather you use anti-inflammatories on your skin, such as aloe vera, panthenol or antibacterials, or use the oils in a soothing diffuser in your room to relax you.

Dr V's Formulation Insights

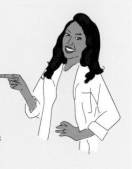

Introducing an allergen to skin of colour doesn't make sense as a rash can lead to hyperpigmentation.

If you are formulating for melanin-rich skin specifically, you wouldn't even have a fragrance or essential oil shelf in your laboratory.

Denatured alcohol

Denatured alcohol is highly volatile and dries the skin. Please read the section on alcohols on page 95.

Contact dermatitis

Contact dermatitis can manifest in different ways and for different reasons.

Irritant contact dermatitis – you may see a red or dark rash with blisters rapidly appear minutes to hours after contact, which makes the cause clear to identify. It occurs due to the concentration of an ingredient and will occur in everyone as it damages the skin barrier.

Allergic contact dermatitis – this takes longer to develop, is not due to concentration of a product and doesn't occur in everyone. It can take weeks or months to develop, in which case the cause isn't always easy to pinpoint. You may just have a mild itch, dry patch or flaking, but it can become exacerbated with each exposure.

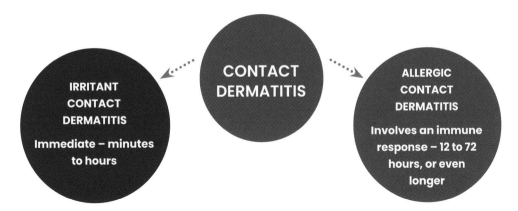

The two most common contact allergens in cosmetics are fragrance and preservatives. This is another reason why I am not a fan of 'natural' ingredients. This is because the preservatives that cause us the *least* amount of contact dermatitis are in fact parabens. I love them and formulate with them. The natural, clean beauty movement demonised them and now a surge of natural preservatives has arisen, which has led to even more contact dermatitis[2] – especially those green products containing Methylisothiazolinone (MIT) and Methylchloroisothiazolinone (MCI).

If you know you are sensitive to products or are just concerned, you can do a patch test to see if you have an allergic reaction to an ingredient, so you will know to avoid it. The main issue is that there are countless fragrances included in skincare, which is why I always recommend fragrance free.

How to recover from contact dermatitis

Contact dermatitis tends to clear up by itself as soon as you remove the irritant. Please look after the skin to avoid breakouts in the first instance and in future avoid fragrances in all cosmetics, and try to avoid scrubbing or scratching your skin. It can take two to three skin-cell cycles to recover, normally about two to three months. In the meantime, use a non-fragrance face wash, moisturiser and SPF50 (mineral, ideally) to create a healing environment for the skin.

Skin friends and skin foes

'I am so confused about all these single ingredient products.'
'What can I combine confidently?'
'Are there actives that if I combine them will lead to sensitivity, irritation or pigmentation?'

Sometimes in our quest to be a best friend to our skin, we end up taking a wrong turn. This chapter will guide you through the combinations that you should avoid at all costs and those that will save you time and money.

What happens when you use a 'bad' combination of ingredients on your skin? The best-case scenario is that you will render the ingredients ineffective as they 'cancel' each other out. In most cases you will see a mild irritation or inflammation, which is a warning sign for you to stop or 'titrate' (slowly increase usage) the ingredients. The worst-case scenario is that inflammatory mediators are released, which trigger the melanocytes and lead to hyperpigmentation in skin of colour.

Here's a quick guide to the most important ingredients to keep apart on your skin:

COMBINATION 1: Ascorbic acid and niacinamide
(This is the most common combination I get asked about by viewers.)

Old research from the 1960s showed that non-stable vitamin C and niacinamide can irritate the skin, but we use stable forms of both now. People also say that combining ascorbic acid and niacinamide converts niacinamide to nicotinic acid. However, this only happens at high temperatures over a long period of time. Our skincare is not subjected to these intense conditions.

Having said this, it is important to know there are many forms of vitamin C, all with different optimal pHs. This is why I would not formulate with ascorbic acid and niacinamide in one cream. I would also avoid layering them, because as we do not absorb 100% of a product, some is left on the surface of the skin and you want each active working at their optimal pHs. I would combine niacinamide with vitamin C derivatives.

Remember. Niacinamide works best from pH 5–7

Ingredient name	Optimal pH	Combines well with niacinamide
Tetrahexyldecyl ascorbate	Oil-soluble and does not have a pH	YES
Sodium ascorbyl phosphate	pH 5.5–7	YES
Magnesium ascorbyl phosphate	pH 5.5–7	YES
Ascorbic acid	pH 3–3.5	NO

COMBINATION 2: Niacinamide and acids (AHA/BHA)

Low-pH acids do not provide an optimal environment for niacinamide to function. Niacinamide is best combined with neutral pH combinations (pH 5–7).

COMBINATION 3: Retinol and exfoliation (physical/chemical)

The vitamin A family (which includes retinol) increases cell turnover rates, so it helps to bring younger skin to the surface. This can lead to dryness and sensitivity, though, so you don't want to further irritate the skin with exfoliation and risk damaging the skin barrier.

COMBINATION 4: Vitamin A and benzoyl peroxide

Benzoyl peroxide actually oxidises retinol and stops it working. It will oxidise all antioxidants including vitamin C, resveratrol and ferulic acid. Benzoyl peroxide is very sensitive and using it at the same time as antioxidants can decrease its effectiveness as an antibacterial.

If you want to use both ingredients for acne, I recommend you apply your benzoyl peroxide, then wait for it to completely dry before applying your antioxidant. Always top off with a fatty, non-fragrance moisturiser with soothing ingredients, such as panthenol or allantoin, to minimise dryness and irritation.

Benzoyl peroxide also inactivates tretinoin (Retin-A), so don't use these at the same time. Retinoid-like compounds, however, such as adapalene, are not affected by benzoyl peroxide.

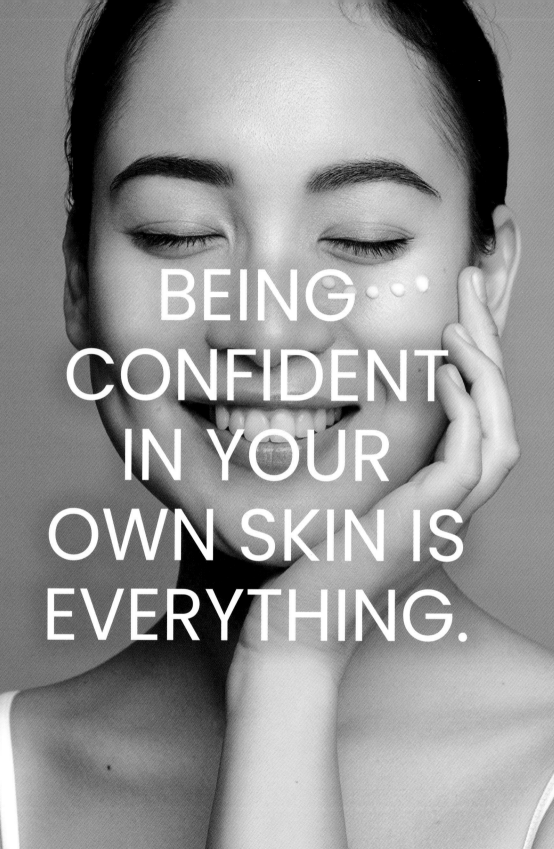

COMBINATION 5: Benzoyl peroxide and exfoliation

Benzoyl peroxide is an antibacterial and clears pores to prevent blocking. I recommend a maximum 2.5% to minimise the chances of irritation.

This is great for treating acne but can lead to dry skin and sensitivity. If the ingredient is too harsh for your skin or the percentage used is too high, you may see flaking. I recommend being gentle with your skin at this point, avoiding exfoliation products, which include glycolic acid and salicylic acid.

> Benzoyl peroxide causes free radicals.
>
> This is a quick reaction and can be countered with antioxidants.
>
> What should you do? Wait 5 minutes AFTER you have applied benzoyl peroxide and apply an antioxidant.

COMBINATION 6: Alcohol toners with any active ingredient afterwards

Denatured alcohol is used for its 'quick-dry' feel, however, it can end up stripping and dehydrating the skin. This impairs the skin barrier, delaying skin repair. It can worsen a lot of skin conditions, including making oily skin even oilier.

Although alcohol does allow more absorption of actives, it can damage skin in the process, so you could end up with more issues, including sensitivity.

COMBINATION 7: Tranexamic acid and low-pH acids

Tranexamic acid works best at a pH of 7. It is mild on the skin and good for skin of colour. Don't use it with other low-pH acids (see below), as it will become less effective if it is not at its optimal pH. This is why a cosmetic formulator would not place these tranexamic acids in the same product as the following low-ph acids:

- Glycolic acid pH 3.5–5
- Salicylic acid pH 2.4
- Lactic acid pH 3–4

COMBINATION 8: Retinol and acids with low pH

Retinol is drying and can be irritating, which is why I don't recommend using it with a low-pH acid.

MYTH: Retinol is an exfoliator.

TRUTH: Not true.

Vitamin A stimulates all cell turnover deep in the skin so that juicy skin cells come to the surface. If you are flaking with vitamin A, it means too much irritation has occurred and, for skin of colour, I would titrate or stop the use of retinol.

By titrate I mean you should start with a small amount and gradually increase it, maybe with short contact one hour a couple nights a week, then wash off. After a few weeks, step up to all night two nights a week. After a few more weeks you may step up to three nights a week. Be gentle with your skin.

Am I purging or breaking out?

'I just started my niacinamide and suddenly I'm breaking out.'
'Everyone loves retinol, why am I breaking out?'
'Am I allergic to salicylic acid, as suddenly I am getting more spots?'

To know if you are purging or breaking out, you need to know what is happening to your skin.

Purging

Purging is when skin cell turnover increases and cells come to the surface faster. This means clogged pores also come to the surface faster so you see a fresh new crop of white heads, black heads and pimples. They were already in the skin and would have shown up in their usual cycle four weeks later, but rapid cell turnover accelerated the process, so you see it all at once.

This is not ideal as it is likely to pigment but the clogged pores resulting in white heads and pimples was likely to happen anyway, only it has just been accelerated as a purge.

Purging can be very frustrating. I often receive DMs from followers who have finally invested time into skin education and money into brand new products, often including vitamin A, only to break out for the first time in years! This can be incredibly disheartening and may even make you stop unless you understand what is happening.

Breakouts

An ingredient is clogging your pores, leading to a plug, which encourages acne to develop. Another thing that might be happening is you could be having a reaction to one of the ingredients. This is a big reason not to change your whole routine all at once.

Ideally, you should introduce only one new ingredient at a time, just once a week, to see how your skin tolerates it, and if there is no detrimental reaction, increase it to two nights a week to allow skin to get used to it.

	Purging	Breakouts
Mechanism of action	Increase cell turnover	Pore-clogging ingredients/ formula
Ingredient examples	BHA/AHAs Retinoids Benzoyl peroxide Exfoliation	Isopropyl myristate Coconut oil Sodium lauryl sulfate Cocoa butter
Duration	4–6 weeks (1 cell cycle)	If it continues for longer than 6 weeks, please discontinue use

For skin of colour, an unnecessary breakout can sometimes mean months of hyperpigmentation to deal with.

How to help your skin recover

Rapid cell turnovers can dry the skin, so to counteract this you need to introduce water magnets (humectants) in your skincare, like sodium hyaluronate, and skin soothers like aloe vera or allantoin.

Are natural products better than synthetic cosmetics?

We have a tendency to think 'natural' means good and 'synthetic' means bad.

This is false information that brands use to sell and take advantage of your desire to treat your skin with care.

Have you ever heard any of these claims?

> Natural is better.
> Natural products are safer as they came from nature.
> Natural products are more sustainable or have higher efficiency.
> Natural products are vegan and cruelty free.
> Natural products contain plant-derived ingredients without harsh chemicals.
> Natural products are clean.
> DIY is best.

Natural is better – first it is important to know that there is no strict definition of 'natural'. If you take it to mean something that is derived from nature, then that includes ingredients such as petroleum jelly used as an occlusive in lip balms, which comes from crude oil originally and then goes through a variety of processes before it becomes petroleum jelly. Some class it as synthetic, others as naturally derived. The same could be said of mandelic acid, which comes from bitter almonds. However, by the time you have the finished ingredient, has it gone through enough chemical processes for it to no longer be considered 'natural'?

On the other hand, we can replicate natural substances in the laboratory that are actually more sustainable and more effective.

Natural products are safer as they came from nature – this is also inaccurate; an example would be essential oils that can sensitise the skin. Fragrance is another good example; this is used in natural deodorants, which can lead to rashes and underarm pigmentation in skin of colour.

I have also seen natural products without preservatives – and these often boast on the label 'no preservatives' – which leads to mould in your skincare products. This is not safe, and in fact if you see this I need you to take your purse and walk in the opposite direction right away.

Remember, 'NAFE is SAFE'.

No
Alcohol (denatured)
Fragrance
Essential oils

Natural products are more sustainable or have higher efficiency – harvesting plants for mass cosmetics manufacturing can be harmful to the planet. There is an assumption that natural is sustainable, but it might not be. Often a huge crop needs to be harvested to extract a very small amount of ingredient. This is a poor return for carbon footprint and for climate change. It is also unnecessarily expensive. To extract rosewood oil, for example, often the entire tree must be cut down. This is unsustainable deforestation. Argan oil has become very popular for hair and skin cosmetics, which is harvested from the *Argania spinosa* tree, which takes 50 years to grow fruit that can be used for its oil. Some sustainable companies give back to the community, but others do not. Having an international carbon footprint rating for ingredients and packaging is currently not standard practice, but I hope in the future this changes.

> *A good product has nothing to do with whether it is derived from nature or synthetically manufactured.*

Natural products are vegan and cruelty free – this is an incorrect assumption. The word natural is an unregulated term and many so-called natural products are not vegan or produced cruelty free.

Natural products contain plant-derived ingredients without harsh chemicals – glycolic acid, my least-favourite AHA for skin of colour, is derived from sugar cane. The acid molecules are tiny and at high percentages can burn and lead to hyperpigmentation. Glycolic acid could be considered a harsh chemical, especially at higher percentages and higher temperatures.

Natural products are clean – this is one that sounds right but is actually a misconception. All cosmetic products are rigorously tested by a third party for safety, microbiology and stability, so how can synthetically derived ingredients be 'dirty'?

DIY is best – DIY facials are so popular and it makes no sense to me. If you don't understand what you are doing and are using inappropriate ingredients there is a high chance of burning and getting hyperpigmentation in skin of colour if you use anything too harsh. I would advise all people with skin of colour to avoid this potentially dangerous practice. It has ruined too many faces.

Lemon juice, apple cider vinegar and whole grains for exfoliation are all big mistakes; honey, yoghurt and eggs are just messy. Plus none of the actives in these ingredients have been calibrated for skin pH. Please avoid.

It is best to have a simple skincare routine of moisturising and using sunscreen than to risk burns and hyperpigmentation from using any of the above. It may have been a good idea for grandparents when they had no other options, but cosmetics have evolved and become more accessible since then.

In case you think I am a 'nature hater', I would like to provide you with a list of natural ingredients that I love in skincare as they have been clinically proven to be effective:

- Oats
- Shea butter
- Glycerin
- Aloe vera
- Jojoba oil
- Bearberry

If you make space for this illogical argument in your mind, you go down a rabbit hole of buying products that don't work or using DIY concoctions that can burn skin of colour. In addition, cosmetic companies will feed off where you are spending your money and will continue to make natural products that give you no indication if they are effective, irritating, sustainable or cost-effective.

Let's stop this cycle by empowering ourselves with knowledge. Just to reinforce my point that I'm not anti-nature – I have also seen excellent ingredient lists on products that have 'natural' being the main marketing message. So, always go further than the marketing and the pretty packaging – ignore the label 'natural' and always thoroughly read the ingredient lists.

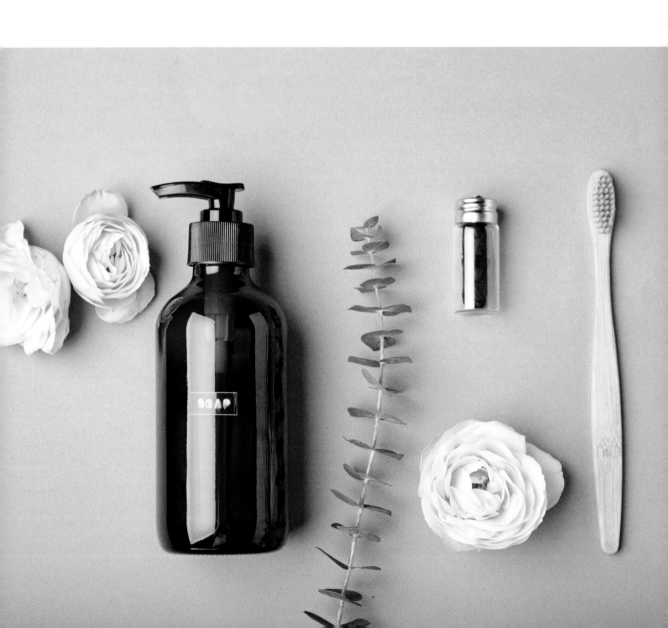

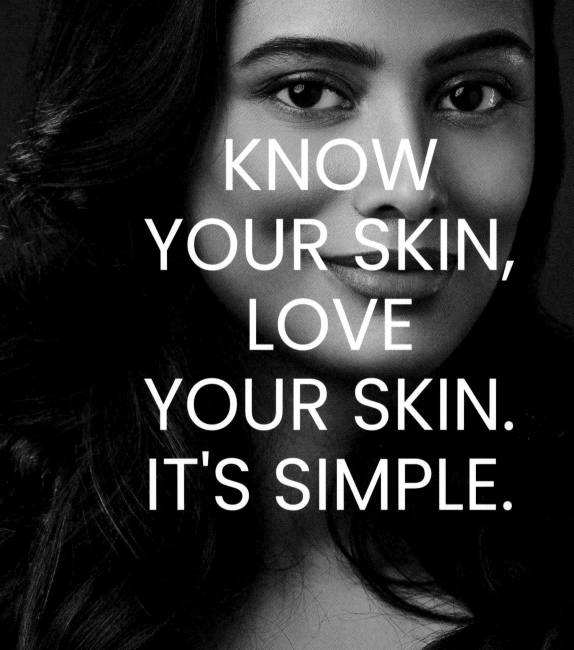

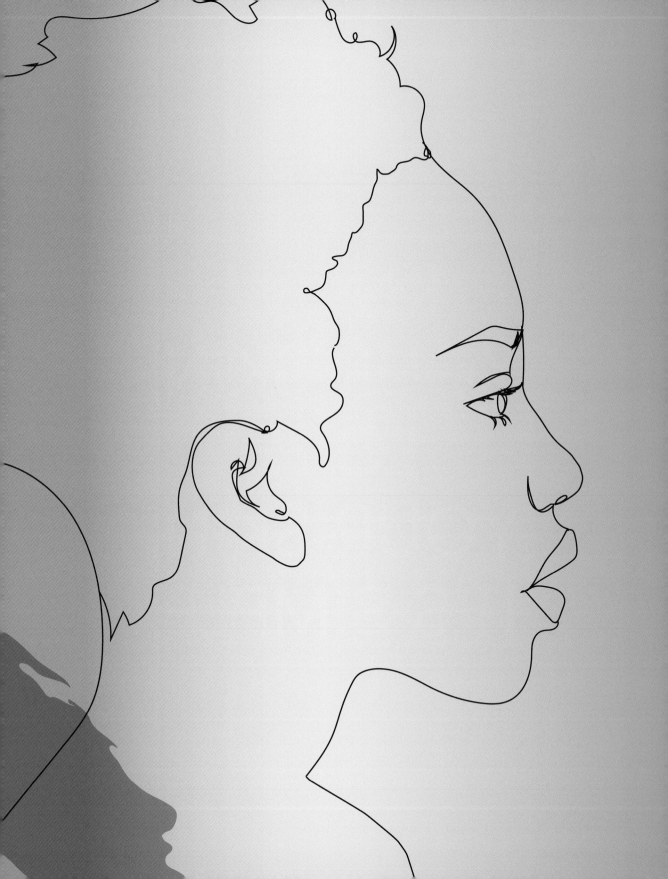

4

How to manage hyper-pigmentation

This chapter will deal with the most common skin problems facing people with skin of colour and arm you with all the knowledge you need to identify and treat these conditions.

I started my discovery journey about hyperpigmentation for skin of colour because once you become a doctor your family starts to ask you about every ailment, and the one question I couldn't answer was 'How do I treat my melasma?' When I looked into it, all the treatments – laser, high-strength TCA/glycolic acid peel and hydroquinone – had side-effects that led to more hyperpigmentation for skin of colour.

It seemed as though these treatments were designed for Caucasian skin, because even if it did cause burns (Fitzpatrick Scale 1–2) it didn't cause more hyperpigmentation. This struck me as incredibly unfair, which sparked my journey trying to walk the fine line of treating hyperpigmentation in skin of colour without burning or leading to more hyperpigmentation.

When I asked my followers how hyperpigmentation impacts their lives, their confidence and ultimately their relationships, I knew I needed to make my Dr V Tyrosinase Inhibiting (Anti-Hyperpigmentation) kits for skin of colour accessible globally.

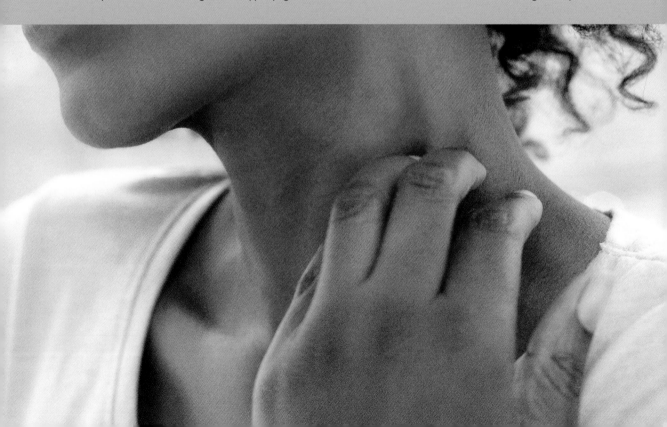

If you have skin of colour and are under 25 years old is addressing hyperpigmentation your biggest concern?

Yes (1766 responses)   **No** (390 responses)

| 82% | 18% |

If you are 25-45 years old with skin of colour is hyperpigmentation your biggest concern?

Yes (3213 responses)   **No** (463 responses)

| 87% | 13% |

If you are 45+ years old with skin of colour is hyperpigmentation your biggest concern?

Yes (967 responses)   **No** (463 responses)

| 77% | 23% |

If you are suffering with hyperpigmentation, does it alter your self-esteem?

Yes (967 responses)   **No** (295 responses)

| 15% | 85% |

What is melasma?

Melasma presents as skin discolouration of the face. Those dark-brown patches often start as innocent freckles in your late twenties and thirties and although people think these freckles are initially 'cute', they are an early warning sign that you are INADEQUATELY protecting your skin from UV damage. Those freckles join up and form patches, they then start to form on other parts of the face.

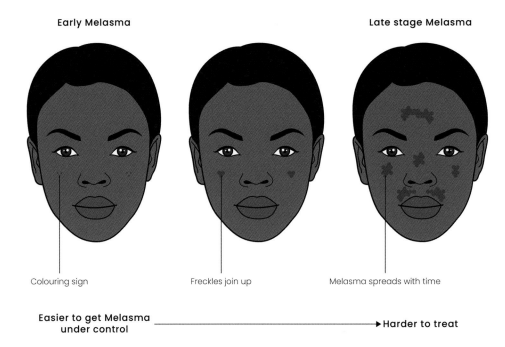

Early Melasma

Late stage Melasma

Colouring sign

Freckles join up

Melasma spreads with time

Easier to get Melasma
under control ──────────────────→ Harder to treat

Usually 80% of melasma starts in the cheekbone area, then spreads to other areas, including the forehead, upper lip and across the nose.

Skin of colour is more likely to suffer from melasma.

There are some additional factors that can influence if you are more prone to melasma:

Genetic factors – if your family has melasma you are more likely to develop it.
UV exposure – years of UV exposure and not wearing SPF50 can be a trigger. This is why we want children to get into the habit of applying SPF50 very early on.
Oestrogen – this is the reason why women are predominantly affected and those with the condition may also find it worsens during pregnancy or from taking the pill, hormone therapy or during the menopause.

During my second pregnancy I was worried about my melasma as I couldn't wear my tyrosinase inhibiting facial kit due to the vitamin A. I used niacinamide, vitamin C and slathered my face with mineral SPF50.

How melasma is formed

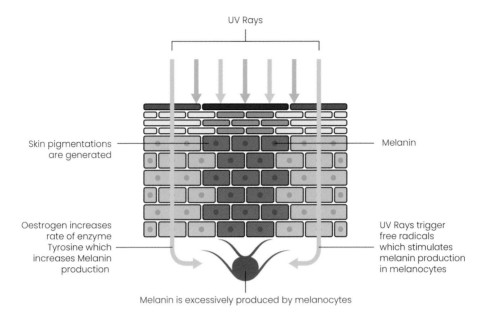

UV Rays

Skin pigmentations are generated

Melanin

Oestrogen increases rate of enzyme Tyrosine which increases Melanin production

UV Rays trigger free radicals which stimulates melanin production in melanocytes

Melanin is excessively produced by melanocytes

How do we treat melasma for skin of colour?

There are professional-grade treatments you can try for your melasma, but if you prefer to give some other options a try first, there are several actives you can use to treat your skin instead.

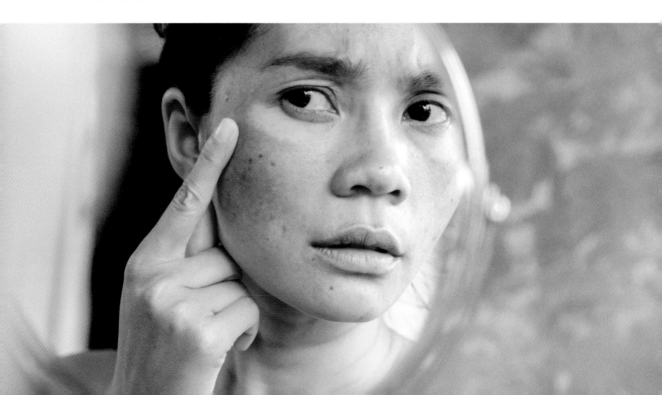

Name of active	How it works
Retinaldehyde	One step removed from retinoic acid. Considered to be more effective than retinol but without the side-effects
Retinol	Two steps removed from retinoic acid. Increases cell turn-over so there is less time for melanin to seep into skin cells
Sodium ascorbyl phosphate	Water-soluble vitamin C (tyrosinase inhibitor and antioxidant)
Ascorbic acid	Water-soluble vitamin C (tyrosinase inhibitor and antioxidant)
Tetrahexyldecyl ascorbate	Fat-soluble vitamin C (tyrosinase inhibitor and antioxidant)
Ferulic acid	Powerful antioxidant
Kojic dipalmitate	Tyrosinase inhibitor
Alpha arbutin	Tyrosinase inhibitor
Octadecenedioic acid	Tyrosinase inhibitor
Liquorice extract	Tyrosinase inhibitor
Phytic acid	Gentle AHA and antioxidant
Niacinamide	Interferes with melanosome transfer, so less melanin moves from melanoctye to skin cells
Azelaic acid	Tyrosinase inhibitor and anti-inflammatory

You will see that tyrosinase inhibitors feature a lot among these actives. However, you are unlikely to see much of a reduction with just 1–2 tyrosinase inhibitors. I prefer using a cocktail of gentle tyrosinase inhibitors to treat hyperpigmentation for skin of colour; they do not burn or lead to PIH for skin of colour when formulated correctly.

Melasma results are completely dependent on wearing SPF50 correctly, large anti-melasma sunglasses and a wide-brimmed hat.

Common mistakes made in treating melasma:

Avoid severe scrubbing. You might think you are removing the top layer of pigmented cells but you may in fact be worsening hyperpigmentation through irritation and any results you think you see are temporary. Your skin is a living organ, so it will grow back. To treat melasma effectively you need to slow the rate of melanin production by using tyrosinase inhibitors.

Avoid irritation or sensitivity from fragrance, alcohol and essential oils as you are already loading the skin with actives at night, so you need to minimise the chances of your skin reacting.

A fatty moisturiser is preferable to use on top, particularly if you have dry skin.

Apply your actives two hours before sleeping so it has time to dry and doesn't come off on your sheets.

You need to reapply your sunscreen every 2–3 hours and avoid direct sunlight. No tyrosinase inhibitors are stronger than the effects of UV on melasma.

Avoid applying any acids during the day.

Please refer to the Tyrosinase Inhibitor section (see page 99) and sunscreen section (see page 66) for my product recommendations.

In one poll I asked:

If you have sensitive skin prone to inflammation, do you prefer mineral sunscreen or chemical?

MINERAL (726 responses)   **CHEMICAL** (193 responses)

| 79% | 21% |

Dr V's Interpretation: In the same poll, 44% of the cohort saw a reduction in melasma when switching from chemical to mineral sunscreen. This is one of the reasons I decided to recommend mineral over chemical for melasma and inflammatory skin conditions.

How can you treat hyperpigmentation?

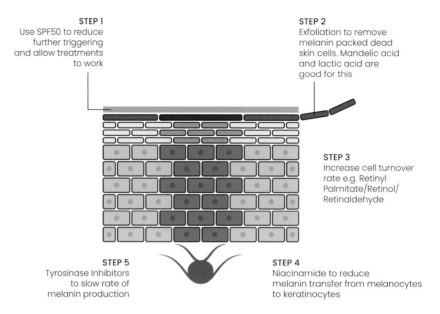

STEP 1
Use SPF50 to reduce further triggering and allow treatments to work

STEP 2
Exfoliation to remove melanin packed dead skin cells. Mandelic acid and lactic acid are good for this

STEP 3
Increase cell turnover rate e.g. Retinyl Palmitate/Retinol/ Retinaldehyde

STEP 4
Niacinamide to reduce melanin transfer from melanocytes to keratinocytes

STEP 5
Tyrosinase Inhibitors to slow rate of melanin production

How can you treat melasma with professional treatments?

There are problems with some professional grade treatments, but here are some options to treat melasma – although not all are ideal for skin of colour.

Laser skin-resurfacing procedures – for darker skin types (Fitzpatrick skin types 3–6) may lead to complications such as hyperpigmentation, hypopigmentation (loss of pigment) and dermal scarring. The dermis is the layer of skin beneath the epidermis and has a rich blood supply, meaning that scarring in this layer of skin can be even more troublesome.

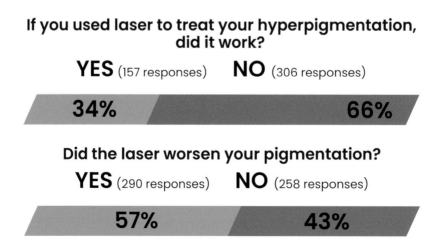

If you used laser to treat your hyperpigmentation, did it work?

YES (157 responses)   **NO** (306 responses)

34%   66%

Did the laser worsen your pigmentation?

YES (290 responses)   **NO** (258 responses)

57%   43%

Microdermabrasion – skin resurfacing is a short-term solution. Skin is a living organ, so just taking off the top layer of dead pigmented skin cells can give a temporary reduction in pigmentation.

If you used microdermabrasion to treat melasma, did it return?

YES (246 responses)   **NO** (132 responses)

65%   **35%**

Chemical peels – I would avoid in particular TCA peels or high-strength glycolic acid. Both can burn the skin and lead to Post-inflammatory Hyperpigmentation (PIH).

Hydroquinone – I am not a fan of this – even though it is the gold standard in treating hyperpigmentation – because of the potential for rebound. Initially you see great results, however, after you stop using it hyperpigmentation often comes back worse than before.

Did you see good results with hydroquinone treating your melasma?

Yes (258 responses)   **No** (478 responses)

| 35% | 65% |

Did your melasma return when you stopped using hydroquinone?

Yes (441 responses)   **No** (122 responses)

| 78% | 22% |

If it returned, was it worse than before?

Yes (280 responses)   **No** (211 responses)

| 57% | 43% |

I know the poll above is likely to be problematic for those who prescribe hydroquinone but polls like this spark change.

Dr V's Interpretation: About 30% of people saw a reduction in the condition with hydroquinone but it has an extremely high recurrence rate of 78%, and the fact it came back worse than before in 57% of people tells me this ingredient is too aggressive for the skin of colour demographic. It appears to further irritate the melanocyte and I would rather you did no treatment than make the situation worse.

MELASMA NEEDS DIFFERENT CARE IN SKIN OF COLOUR.

Dark circles

'What are dark circles and why do they happen?'
'Can hereditary dark circles be treated?

Dark circles around the eyes tend to appear after puberty, from 16 to 25 years old. They are more common in skin of colour. Don't confuse dark circles (known as periorbital pigmentation) with eye bags – the latter is a mild swelling or puffiness under the eyes that happens later in life due to laxity of skin and muscles in this area.

A study on 209 candidates in the Indian *Journal of Dermatology* showed 47.5% of participants had periorbital pigmentation, aka dark circles, and 63% of those who had this had a family history of it, so were classed as 'hereditary pigmentation'.

The main causes of dark circles are:

- Hyperpigmentation – hyperactive melanocytes around the eye area.
- Volume loss – can lead to shadowing, which appears as dark circles.
- Venous pooling from allergies can give the appearance of dark circles.

The majority of creams will not work, such as using a caffeine cream to constrict blood vessels, nor a niacinamide cream or a few antioxidants. This is because periorbital pigmentation is one of the most stubborn forms of pigmentation, and one that has often been there for decades.

You need a number of different high-strength actives to target periorbital pigmentation.

What is happening on a cellular level?

Skin of colour tends to have large melanocytes clustered around the eye area. They are easily triggered and produce too much pigment, therefore you need tyrosinase inhibitors. Dark circles worsen with age as the skin around the eyes thins. We need to improve skin texture and elasticity, too, which is why you also need to boost collagen and hydration levels.

Hereditary dark circles can be treated

Having hereditary dark circles just means you have a tendency for melanocytes to over-produce melanin. You can still use actives to decrease the rate of melanin production, it may take longer and be more stubborn, but you can improve it, as it is still just hyperpigmentation (especially if it is epidermal pigmentation).

What ingredients are needed to treat dark circles?

Vitamin A – one of my favourite forms of vitamin A is retinyl palmitate for around the eye, as the skin around the eye is about 0.3mm thick. Retinyl palmitate increases cell turnover, so younger cells come to the surface faster. It also improves skin texture and mops up free radicals, which leads to premature ageing.

Vitamin C (Sodium ascorbyl phosphate) – water-soluble vitamin C interacts with copper ions on the enzyme tyrosinase, slowing the rate of melanin production.

Vitamin C (Tetrahexyldecyl ascorbate) – fat-soluble vitamin C penetrates the dermis to help restore collagen. Dark circles worsen with age as collagen is destroyed and skin appears thinner. We need to improve the texture and structure of the skin to decrease the appearance of dark circles.

Vitamin E (Tocopherol acetate) – antioxidants work best in combination, and using vitamins E and C together is an excellent option.

Niacinamide – slows the rate of melanosomes from melanocytes transferring to the surrounding skin cells, which results in seeing less hyperpigmentation on the surface.

Key tyrosinase inhibitors:

Kojic acid dipalmitate – the best form of kojic acid for the eye area for skin of colour. It inhibits melanin production without irritating the skin.

Alpha arbutin – this is an effective tyrosinase inhibitor with very little irritation. Works well in combination with other tyrosinase inhibitors.

Octadecenedioic acid – this is more effective than azelaic acid with little to no irritation. A study of 96 Mexican females of 1% octadecenedioic acid (aka. dioic acid) vs 2% HQ saw equal reduction of pigmentation by 40% after 12 weeks but with very few side-effects.

Liquorice extract – excellent as a skin brightener. Glabidin is a component of liquorice, which is an antioxidant and skin soother.

Urva-ursi extract – a powerful antioxidant and tyrosinase inhibitor.

Moisturisers – Sodium hyaluronate, glycerine, urea, lactic acid – the skin around the eye area tends to get fine lines first. We improve this by increasing the hydration levels of the epidermis. One molecule of hyaluronic acid draws many molecules of water like a water magnet to plump the skin.

Emollients – Cetearyl alcohol, Simmondsia seed oil, Parkii (shea) butter – emollients smooth the edges of skin cells so they reflect light evenly, giving you translucent skin.

Anti-inflammatory – Allantoin, aloe, panthenol – to soothe the skin as you are using many actives on thin, sensitive, delicate skin.

Lip hyperpigmentation

The lip colour you are born with is your natural lip colour. However, darkening can happen due to the following reasons:

- Smoking
- UV-induced lip pigmentation
- Trauma

- Injury
- Inflammation from cosmetics, irritating acids or spices in food

Inflammation ·····▷ Triggers Melanocyte-stimulating hormone (MSH) ·····▷ Increased melanin production

Lips have a very thin epidermis of 3–5 cells compared to the cheeks, which are about 16 cells thick. The thin tissue of the lips mean that the blood vessel colour is shown as 'pink lips'. This is why you can't use the same treatment for facial hyperpigmentation as for lip hyperpigmentation.

Mistakes I have seen being made include: Laser, IPL or Cryotherapy to treat lip hyperpigmentation for skin of colour. These treatments can lead to irritation and more hyperpigmentation.

Some people are also fed up with this cycle:

Lipstick causes lip pigmentation

Wear more lipstick to 'hide the lip pigmentation'

So they just get a lip tattoo, but this has its own issues. Not only does the treatment need to be repeated every few years, it's painful, and there is also a risk of minor side-effects including minor erythema, infection, rashes or scars.

Stopping the trigger is essential for hyperpigmentation. Usually you would need to:

- Quit smoking.
- Wear SPF30–50 lip balm throughout the day.
- Avoid daily matte lipsticks. Stick with petroleum jelly to lock in hydration.
- If you have eaten fruit acids or ginger during the day, wash your lips and apply your SPF50 lip balm.

Dr V's Formulation Insights

I conducted a clinical trial when trying to find a way of treating lip hyperpigmentation without leading to irritation and more hyperpigmentation. This was a delicate balance as the skin on the lips is so thin.

After many failed attempts I opted to try a tyrosinase inhibiting scrub to remove the top layer of pigmented skin cells and improve penetration of actives. I originally tried using a chemical exfoliator but this yielded poor results due to poor compliance – because the taste was terrible! It is just as important to look at the response of users in these trials as it is to look at the effects of the formula.

I then decided to follow up with the tyrosinase inhibiting mask and balm to lock in the actives.

After formulating, you really should conduct an independent clinical study on your ideal cohort to see if it actually works. There is no point otherwise. This is the scariest part for me; imagine having invested years of your life and a bottomless pit of resources to create a product, only for it to be completely out of your hands when you send it off for clinical trials? I wrote the three-month results due date in my diary and tried to continue with my life.

Every time clinical results come back I would get a huge brief with tables and charts. I'd hunt through the pages looking for the only bit of information I needed … did it work or not?

It would send me reeling back to my GCSE results at 16 years old scouring for a 'B' which meant I probably wouldn't get into medical school and that my Indian immigrant parents would very likely proceed to disown me (sorry, that took a dark turn – remnants of my childhood trauma!).

When the LipX kit results came back I actually jumped up and down, squealing with happiness and pride. My husband came running in thinking something terrible had happened but I leapt on the poor unsuspecting man and made him topple backwards! Those amazing results that day were that 100% of our LipX candidates had seen a reduction in lip hyperpigmentation, which was unheard of in a clinical trial.

Actives I recommend to treat lip hyperpigmentation:

Tyrosinase inhibitors – to decrease the rate of melanin production.

Retinyl palmitate – (correct vitamin A for lips) as this is less likely to dry them but will increase cell turnover.

Kojic dipalmitate – a more stable and less irritating form of kojic acid.

Alpha arbutin – a very powerful tyrosinase inhibitor that is suitable for skin of colour and works well in combination with other tyrosinase inhibitors; 2% is the ideal percentage.

Azeloglycline – Azelaic acid and 10% glycerin is the ideal percentage for lips in skin of colour. It's an excellent tyrosinase inhibitor but has low irritation due to the moisturising effect of glycerine.

Niacinamide – reduces the rate of melanosome packets travelling to surrounding cells. There is no irritation, which is great for skin of colour.

Octadecanedioic acid– reduces stress-induced hyperpigmentation and melanin transfer to skin cells.

Tocopheryl acetate – vitamin E mops up free radicals that stimulate pigmentation.

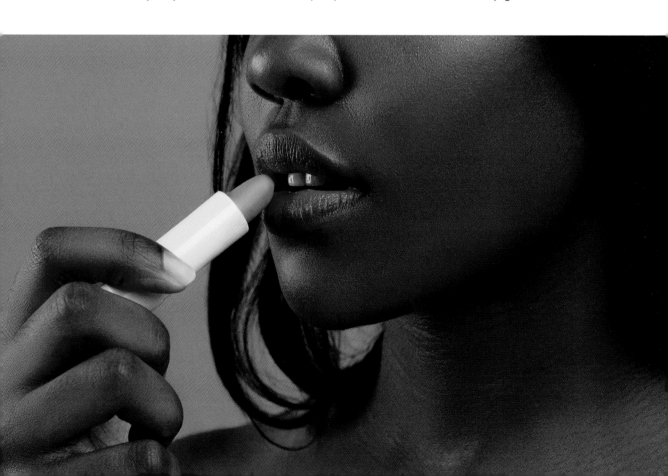

Dark knees and elbows

About 10% of those who have visited me at my hyperpigmentation clinic arrive with complaints about 'dark knees' and 'dark elbows'. This can stop people from wearing clothes that expose these areas and is an unwanted aesthetic that can feel very restrictive at times.

Dark knees and elbows are also known as 'frictional asymptomatic darkening of extensor surfaces'. The hyperpigmentation is symmetrical, and no pain is experienced. It tends to start during puberty and can worsen after friction, as the medical name suggests – such as housework, construction or praying on your knees daily. This chronic friction can lead to inflammation, which triggers the melanocytes and leads to more pigmentation.

Friction also thickens the skin, which means that the worst thing you can do is try to scrub your skin. The top layer of dead skin cells will be temporarily removed but your skin is a living organ, so the cells will grow back. You would need to:

- Block the trigger – stop the friction, don't kneel for long periods.
- Use tyrosinase inhibitors.
- Block further UV stimulation by using broad-spectrum SPF50 – especially when exposed.

Ingredients to use at night on affected areas:

Melanosome transfer disruption:

2–5% niacinamide

Antioxidants:

Vitamin C
Vitamin E

Ferulic acid antioxidants
Resveratrol

Tyrosinase inhibitors:

Kojic acid or kojic dipalmitate
Alpha arbutin
Green tea extract

Liquorice root extract
Bearberry

Moisturise:

Fatty, non-fragranced moisturiser.

During the day:

Broad spectrum SPF50. I prefer zinc oxide for its anti-inflammatory properties.

Worst DIY mistakes

I first started sharing my knowledge about skin online – with my medical background and experience as a formulator – as I knew a lot of people had been burnt following online DIY advice. Some of these videos posted online had had millions of views, which made me wonder how many people had also burnt their skin trying that advice?

Classic DIY mistakes include:

Self-made physical scrubs with crushed nut shells or whole grains

Lemon juice with a low pH

Apple cider vinegar

Garlic

Avocado oil

Inner-thigh darkening

This is another condition I see a lot in the clinic, usually in the run up to summer when people know they will soon be showing more skin. This is mainly a condition that affects skin of colour. A study in 2007[3] confirmed darkening of skin (dyschromia) to be the second most common diagnosis of Black American patients, but even so it didn't make it into the top 19 most common diagnoses for Caucasian patients.

The condition occurs because when inner thighs rub together, friction develops creating thermal energy (heat). This results with inflammation, which releases a whole host of chemicals in your skin – prostaglandins, cytokines and reactive oxygen species. These all stimulate melanin production from your melanocytes.

Friction ·····> Inflammation ·····> Pigmentation

How to treat it

The first thing to do is to stop the root cause: friction. Nothing else will help if this is not addressed. So, wear trousers or cycling shorts underneath your skirt or dust your skin with talcum powder where your thighs meet.

Key ingredients for products

Retinoids **–** increase cell turnover, giving less time for melanosomes (melanin parcels) to seep into surrounding skin cells.

I prefer to use a cream or serum that combines:

0.3% retinol for the body

Retinaldehyde (usually formulated at less than 0.05% but can be formulated up to 0.1%)

Encapsulated retinol (usually formulated up to 2%)

The following ingredients are usually found in single quantities or in combinations of two or three. For skin of colour I prefer using most of these in a cocktail cream.

Azelaic acid 10–20%
Kojic dipalmitate
Alpha arbutin 2%
2–5% niacinamide with N-acetylglucosamine

Ascorbic acid is an antioxidant and tyrosinase inhibitor. It is an unstable ingredient and degrades in oxygen. We can put it through a chemical reaction to create a more stable, less irritating derivative, such as sodium ascorbyl phosphate.

Liquorice extract contains glabridin, which inhibits tyrosinase and has anti-inflammatory properties that can help with PIH especially.

Common mistakes:

If you are too harsh with treating inner thigh darkening, you will worsen the pigmentation. Melanocytes are unpredictable in skin of colour. Always choose the non-irritating option or you run the risk of making the pigmentation darker and more resistant.

Product suggestions:

Please refer to the tyrosinase inhibitor section on page 99.

Hyperpigmentation around the mouth area

It is important to understand the cause of your hyperpigmentation before you can choose the best way to manage it. Hyperpigmentation around the mouth area has two main causes.

Around the mouth hyperpigmentation

Hormonal   Inflammatory

Hormonal causes

It is common for women in our skin-of-colour family to suddenly develop hyperpigmentation around the mouth area during puberty. Women learn to colour-correct this area before applying makeup and use shades of foundation that work well for the rest of the face, but this can make this area look ashy. This diffuse hyperpigmentation can cover the upper lip, sides of the mouth and come down to the chin.

Inflammatory causes

Mouth hyperpigmentation can occur because of:

Eczema

Contact dermatitis

The corners of the lips becoming dry and leading to sore, flaking skin (angular cheilitis)

Managing hormonal and inflammatory mouth hyperpigmentation requires slowing down the rate of the enzyme tyrosinase, which is responsible for producing melanin.

Key ingredients for products

Please wear your actives at night to allow them to work without the negative effect of elements from the environment. There are some specific actives that I recommend.

To reduce the amount of melanin coming to the surface of the hyperpigmented area:

2–5% niacinamide

Antioxidants:

Vitamin C

Vitamin E

Ferulic acid antioxidants

Resveratrol

Tyrosinase inhibitors:

Kojic acid or kojic dipalmitate

Alpha arbutin

Green tea extract

Liquorice root extract

Bearberry

Moisturiser:

Fatty, non-fragranced moisturiser

Broad spectrum SPF50 mineral during the day

MYTH: When you tan, your hyperpigmentation appears less obvious.

TRUTH: When you tan your skin is darkening and your hyperpigmentation is being camouflaged. When you lose the tan, your hyperpigmented patch has often darkened further. Tanning is a temporary measure that actually ages the skin and stimulates your melanocytes further.

> **A potential routine for treating mouth hyperpigmentation is:**
>
> 5–10% niacinamide – The Ordinary, Paula's Choice, Naturium, Be Minimalist (£)
>
> 3% resveratrol + 3% ferulic – The Ordinary (£)
>
> 2% alpha arbutin – The Ordinary, Naturium (£)
>
> Moisturise with F Balm Drunk Elephant, Cetraben or Cerave (££)

Dr V's Formulation Insights

Mouth hyperpigmentation is almost as stubborn to treat as dark circle hyperpigmentation. I had to incorporate 12 actives into the Facial Pigmentation Kit and still only started seeing results for pigmentation in this area after six months.

The reason is that you are likely to have had the hyperpigmentation for over a decade by the time you do treatment, which contributes to stubbornness of the pigmentation.

How do you manage inflammatory mouth hyperpigmentation?

'Dermatitis' means inflamed skin. There are many causes of inflammation, and in skin of colour it triggers the melanocytes leading to more pigmentation.

Contact dermatitis – the key here is to block the trigger. If inflammation is caused by contact dermatitis, make sure you have no fragrance, essential oils or drying alcohol in your skincare products. It may also occur from spices and fruit acids that have not been removed from the skin properly, especially if you then go out into the sun. Examples of known irritating foods, spices and fruits include cinnamon, ginger, oranges, pineapples and mangos.

Eczema – if the cause is eczema, you MUST repair the damaged skin barrier to prevent more TEWL. Increased water evaporation means the skin is not functioning optimally, then irritants and bacteria can enter the skin, leading to further inflammation and more water evaporation. This leads to pain, itching, bleeding and even secondary infections. The key is to use very thick occlusives, such as petrolatum, to behave as a second skin, locking water in. (See chapter seven on Ezcema.)

Angular chelitis – this is when the corners of the lips feel dry and you keep licking them. This further dehydrates the skin and leads to more irritation. The key here is to stop licking and carry a non-fragrance petroleum lip balm – like original Vaseline. Apply this 5–10 times a day to keep skin feeling comfortable, supple and hydrated.

Cracking of skin in this area will only lead to more pigmentation, which is difficult to treat because of the location of the broken skin.

Underarm hyperpigmentation

I classically see this condition in my clinic during wedding season, as many people are uncomfortable wearing sleeveless tops while having underarm pigmentation.

The problem with underarm hyperpigmentation is that is where the skin is thin and there tends to be a lot of friction as it is a 'fold' and it heats up fast, which increases how rapidly the acids penetrate the skin.

There's nothing more irritating than inflamed underarms! I had a bad experience with a new natural deodorant that made my underarms so itchy and red that they became sensitive. It took two weeks for my skin barrier to recover.

When I bothered to read the ingredients (instead of just trusting a friend's recommendation!), I couldn't believe how loaded with fragrance the product was, they started from the fourth ingredient – a high percentage. This product also had sodium bicarbonate as the first ingredient. When this ingredient is used in small amounts it is fine, but used as the first ingredient it is at a very high percentage, and being alkaline it stripped the skin's oil barrier, which is meant to remain acidic. This is just one example of how easy it is to get irritated and sensitised underarm skin that can potentially lead to hyperpigmentation.

Typical causes and triggers of underarm hyperpigmentation

- Classically, you see this during puberty in skin of colour. Simultaneously, hyperpigmentation develops around the mouth and groin area. The cause here is hormonal and mostly affects women.

- Inflammation, such as eczema, skin infections and contact dermatitis.

- Another common cause is Acanthosis nigricans. This is seen as thickened, 'velvety' skin that affects the folds, including underarms, neck and groin. (See page 206 for more information on this condition.)

To treat underarm hyperpigmentation, you must always stop the trigger first. You can do this in a few ways once you have determined the cause:

- Improve the dry, broken skin barrier if the cause is eczema.

- If the cause is Acanthosis nigricans, reduce the amount of sugar in your diet to control blood glucose levels.

- Treat any skin infections, if this is the cause.

- Make sure you stop using irritating ingredients or products if they are triggering the pigmentation.

Common mistakes:

People feel that scrubbing this area lightens the hyperpigmentation, but the problem is you are just temporarily removing of the top layer of pigmented skin cells and can also further trigger melanocytes so pigmentation returns and may spread. It's better to use a chemical exfoliation like mandelic acid.

Two other common causes of underarm PIH include:

Shaving – avoid nickel razor blades if you have an allergy. Ensure you use a fragrance-free shaving cream and replace blades regularly so they are sharp and you avoid tugging or repeating an area.

Deodorants – avoid natural deodorants, as they often contain irritating ingredients.

Additional ingredients I recommend as skin soothers if you suffered with underarm irritation:

- Green tea extract
- Allantoin
- D-panthenol
- *Centella Asiatica*

To ease the irritation caused by PIH in the underarm, follow this simple daily routine:

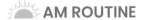 ## AM ROUTINE

Step 1: Wash with an unfragranced gentle wash.
Step 2: Apply a hypo-allergenic deodorant.
Step 3: If your underarm is going to be exposed to sunlight, apply your SPF50.

🌙 PM ROUTINE

Step 1: Wash with an unfragranced gentle wash
Step 2: Apply tyrosinase inhibitors and skin soothers (please read the Tyrosinase Inhibitor section on page 99 for product recommendations).
Step 3: Finish with a fatty moisturiser.

The reason why I decided to learn how to formulate for skin of colour was because I was hearing comments just like this:

'I was surprised to learn that a common side-effect of the classic hyperpigmentation treatments included inflammation or burns, which led to more hyperpigmentation.'

It struck me as odd that nobody had thought this was a potential problem. Classic hyperpigmentation treatments include laser, TCA peels or high-strength glycolic acid and hydroquinone (see page 124). The majority of these treatments were discovered and designed in the west for Caucasian skin, which have smaller and less-reactive melanin-producing cells and fewer melanin parcels (melanosomes) per cell. This then became the classic 'hyperpigmentation playbook' for the rest of the world.

Unfortunately, these treatments can burn skin of colour and lead to more pigmentation. I conducted a series of polls on my Instagram page to see how widespread the issue of hyperpigmentation was for skin of colour, and these were the responses.

Laser treatment

If you used laser to treat hyperpigmentation, did it work?

YES (158 responses)　　**NO** (284 responses)

34%	66%

Did laser worsen the hyperpigmentation?

YES (290 responses)　　**NO** (218 responses)

57%	43%

To have 57% of 509 of people with skin of colour get more pigmentation after laser indicates to me that the side effects are NOT worth doing this treatment.

Dr V's Formulation Insights

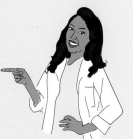

When formulating for skin of colour you must ask these two questions in the CORRECT order:

1. What will cause the *least* amount of irritation?

2. What will give me the most effective formulation?

Unfortunately, company questions tend to be:

1. How do I create a marketable product (even if it might not be in the therapeutic range as we do not need to disclose efficacy?)

2. How do I make the product as cheap as possible to produce and sell?

Rarely is the question about irritation even asked – unless for an eczema product.

The cosmeceutical world is not transparent. We are dependent on the marketing and how expensive an advert looks, which has zero to do with what is in a product. I have analysed very expensive skincare products that claim to be 'anti-ageing' but not only have zero anti-ageing ingredients but are actually loaded with skin sensitisers and dehydrating ingredients – the exact opposite of what ageing skin requires. Always look beyond the marketing and study the ingredients list.

Step-by-step – what to do if your skin burns

In this situation, to ease your skin you want your blood vessels to constrict quickly to stop inflammation-causing mediators flooding the burnt area. How do you do this? To cool the area rapidly, apply a cloth soaked in cold running water or a wrapped-up ice pack. Do this for 5–20 minutes until the inflammation has stopped.

Inflammatory mediators trigger your melanocytes leading to hyperpigmentation. A common mistake is to use a healing 'balm' immediately, but as they retain heat, they will not cool down the burnt area.

Please avoid any products with fragrance, denatured alcohol or essential oils.

You may be able to purchase 1% hydrocortisone over the counter or get a prescription from your doctor to use for a week or two, which will further reduce inflammation.

Once the inflammation has gone down, apply an aloe soothing gel 3–4 times a day. After that, switch to a fattier, non-fragranced moisturiser. You need to moisturise 3–4 times a day to ensure the skin is hydrated, which creates a 'healing' environment.

After a week or two, hyperpigmentation may set in despite your best efforts to reduce inflammation. You need to start using tyrosinase inhibitors at this point. (Please read the tyrosinase inhibiting section on page 99.)

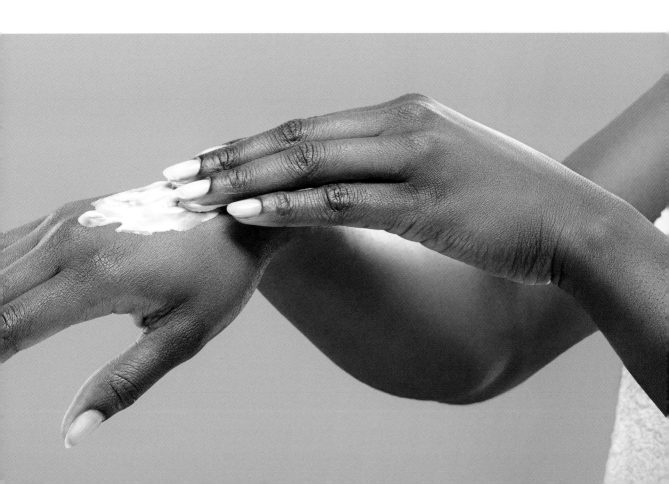

Worst DIY hyperpigmentation mistakes

A beautiful young lady walked in to my clinic once with a huge black burn mark across her face. She was distressed and I couldn't think what had caused the mark. I wish I could say it was the last time I ever saw something similar.

This young lady had been watching YouTube videos on how to clear blemishes. She followed someone who told her to use apple cider vinegar on the face. This is disastrous because the pH of apple cider vinegar is 2–3 and the pH of skin is 4.5–6.5 and is not equipped to tolerate such a low pH. As a result, apple cider vinegar burns the skin and our large, sensitive melanocytes kick into gear, spitting out extra melanin in anger. Our melanoctyes do not tolerate any form of inflammation.

Hearing this, was the exact moment I decided to create my YouTube channel to explain what we can and can't do to our skin, based on first-hand clinical data.

The other phrase I often hear is:

'If it is good enough to eat, it is good enough to put on my skin.'

The stomach contains gastric acid, it is designed for low pH of 1–3, which is needed when you are breaking down protein and digesting your food. Your skin, however, can't tolerate low pH, and any irritation from an extremely acidic substance damages the skin barrier. This leads to more TEWL, and as a result your blood vessels expand and inflammatory mediators flood the affected area, which leads to dryness, redness or darkening of, or peeling of the skin. This inflammation can then trigger your melanocytes, which can cause PIH (Post-inflammatory hyperpigmentation, see page 171 for more on this).

I have also seen upper lip burns from people using ginger and potato on their skin, as well as from TCA peels purchased online. These are just a few examples, and there are many more below.

Lemon juice – this is the number one culprit. A client was following a trusted lifestyle influencer who demonstrated how she used lemon juice to brighten her skin. My client proceeded to do the same, but this damaged her skin barrier, which led to redness, then hyperpigmentation. Thankfully we treated the skin in time so there was no long-lasting damage. However, this is a common mistake, and without intervention it can leave you with a lifetime of hyperpigmentation.

People think lemon juice is great as the vitamin C and citric acid it contains brightens and exfoliates dead skin, but in fact it does more harm than good.

In addition, inflammation can occur when citrus sits on the skin during the day if you are out in the sun with UV rays on your face, which may present as redness or burgundy colour, swelling and blistering. This is why you should always wash your lips after eating citric fruit, especially in the sun.

Note: Citric acid used to buffer a cream is not at a high enough percentage to cause a reaction.

Scrubbing with whole grains – this is another common problem. I did a reaction video to some celebrities on YouTube who show their 'homemade' skincare routines, and this was one of the worst ingredients used.

Whole grains are uneven, have sharp edges and can lead to micro tears of the skin, because it is an uncontrolled ingredient. This damages the skin barrier, leading to redness or burgundy colour, irritation, breakouts and sensitivity.

Garlic – I have seen a patient in my clinic who thought using garlic on the upper lip would improve melasma. Unfortunately, garlic is another natural ingredient that can lead to chemical burns, leading to more hyperpigmentation.

The main chemical ingredient in garlic that causes these burns is diallyl disulfide. This can cause contact dermatitis and rashes.

Apple cider vinegar for acne – the process of fermenting apple cider to make vinegar gives the finished product a low pH, and it contains both malic acid and citric acid at high concentrations. So unfortunately, apple cider vinegar is very acidic and can cause burns when applied directly to skin.

Final thoughts on DIY hyperpigmentation treatments

The risk/reward ratio doesn't work in your favour. You need to use tyrosinase inhibitors at the correct percentages, formulated in the right way, to effectively reduce the rate of melanin production.

The best you can achieve with DIY treatments is to strip away the top layer of skin, which any scrub can do. I am not a fan of scrubs to exfoliate skin of colour, as you aren't just removing the top layer of dead skin cells but potentially causing other problems (see exfoliation section on page 47).

HEALTHY AND HAPPY SKIN CAN BE YOURS WHEN YOU KNOW HOW TO HEAL IT.

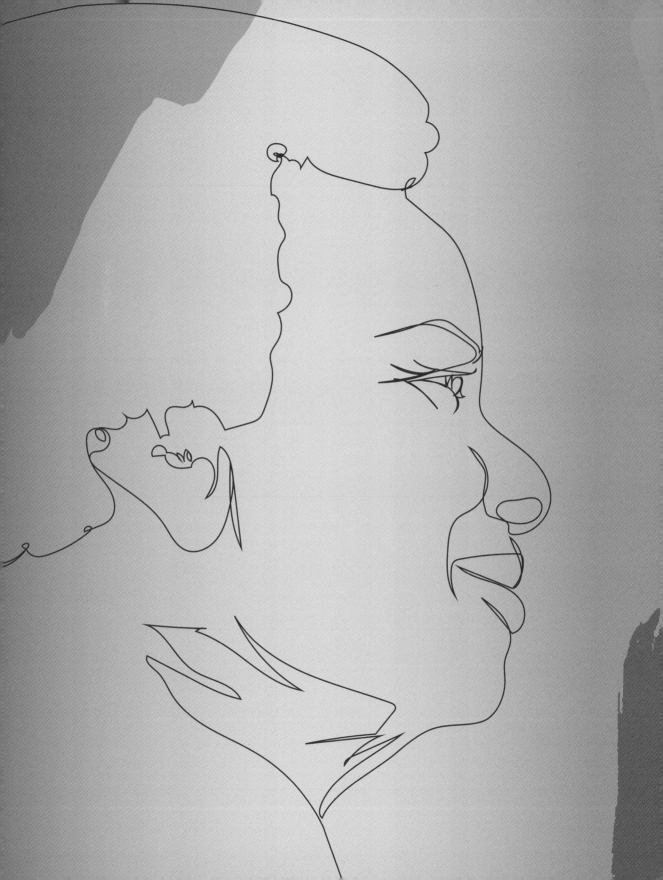

5

Skincare throughout your LIFETIME

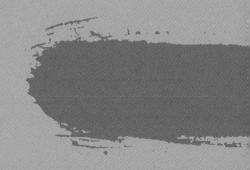

If you are reading this section, it is because you really want to know what is going on with this new, stubborn, deep-set wrinkle on your face that you don't particularly want to see.

This is a huge topic, and one that does not get enough attention in online skincare advice, but that affects us all from our early thirties. I want to explain the ageing process in skin properly so you are empowered moving forward and you know exactly why you need to complete each step in your anti-ageing routine.

This part of the book is your guide to achieving that youthful glow we're all chasing, and in the following pages we will cover:

- Why skin ages and what you can do about it.
- The single biggest cause of premature ageing skin and how to reverse it.
- What skincare ingredients and step-by-step routine you require.

Why skin ages and what you can do about it

Issue 1: Hormonal changes

When your period stops during menopause, there is a reduction in testosterone, oestrogen and sex-hormone binding proteins. Oestrogen stimulation increases the amount of glucosaminoglycans (the water magnets in our skin), one of which is hyaluronic acid.

Hyaluronic acid is important in skin because it acts like a water magnet to create a gel-like substance that fills the space between collagen and elastin fibres in the dermis.

Water in the epidermis hydrates and plumps the skin, giving you juicy looking skin with light reflecting evenly off the flawless surface. This is how you can get the mystical glow we all want.

Producing less hyaluronic acid will mean more water evaporating from our skin (TEWL), which is why skin feels dry and dull as we age. Skin can age rapidly, resulting in more wrinkles, dryness, decreased firmness, thickness and elasticity.

Solution: This is why humectants in skincare are essential, such as hyaluronic acid, urea and glycerine in anti-ageing skincare.

Issue 2: Loss of collagen

Collagen is a structural protein that provides strength to the dermis.

> *Age reduces the rate of collagen formation and accelerates the rates of breakdown. It's a double whammy.*

As it decreases, it leads to wrinkling and sagging – all of our favourite things!

Solution: Thankfully, there are five solutions to this issue:

- Collagen stimulation with tetrahexyldecyl ascorbate (fat-soluble vitamin C).
- Retinaldehyde (more effective and less irritating than retinol) and peptides.
- Controlled microneedling is a good option.
- Drinking marine collagen is a great supplement if you eat less protein than your daily requirement. Skin is considered the 'least important organ of the body' and protein will be used by all other organs first.

Dr V's Formulation Insights

What do you microneedle with for a deep wrinkle?

As we do not know the exact percentage of vitamin A being converted and effectively used as retinoic acid, for a deep wrinkle I recommend using a product with all three over-the-counter vitamin As, including retinyl palmitate (naturally found in our body), retinol 0.1% (can be irritating and if you microneedle with it, keep the percentage low) and retinaldehyde (one step removed from retinoic acid).

I would also use the other two actives known to stimulate collagen with minimal irritation – tetrahexyldecyl ascorbate and peptides.

Even though glycolic acid does stimulate collagen production, I wouldn't dermaroll with it as it would be far too irritating.

Please read the microneedling section on page 219.

Issue 3: More reactive skin that takes longer to recover

The reduction in concentration of fats can create a drier skin and a less protective skin barrier. This reduces the epidermal barrier function.

Solution: The last stage of a skincare routine, when you are post menopause, should be a facial oil, to trap water molecules in the skin – especially if you use heating or air conditioning!

Issue 4: Increased hyperpigmentation

The number of melanocytes decrease as you age, but the remaining ones increase in size. This is why the skin looks paler, with large, pigmented spots.

Solution: Tyrosinase inhibitors are essential as part of your skincare routine.

It is important to know that ageing is due to multiple causes and needs a multi-pronged defensive strategy, in your skincare and your lifestyle. Premature ageing is caused by both intrinsic and extrinsic factors.

Intrinsic factors – genes control our natural ageing process and are referred to as the intrinsic factor. This accounts for 10% of the ageing process and it starts to show after 60 years of age.

Extrinsic factors – those that come from outside the body. They account for 90% of the ageing process and are environmental- and lifestyle-dependent. One of the biggest environmental causes of ageing is free radicals. Free radicals are extremely reactive atoms or molecules that attack collagen, elastin and, worst of all, our DNA (this is what causes skin cancers, for example). The most common causes of free radicals are:

UV radiation

Air pollution

Alcohol

Smoking

What can you do to decrease the risk of free radicals and premature ageing?

Use sunscreen (decrease free radicals from all UV damage)

Use antioxidants on your skin

Reduce inflammation

Reduce stress

Antioxidants

Skin is constantly being damaged from UV rays in our daily life. Antioxidants neutralise free radicals, reducing damage from the sun's radiation. You can introduce antioxidants to your body either topically from skincare or directly from food.

Skincare antioxidants

Think **ACE:**
Vitamins **A**, **C** and **E** are key for anti-ageing.

To this, I would add green tea extract, liquorice extract, ferulic acid and niacinamide as other amazing antioxidants. We need both water-soluble antioxidants, such as vitamins A and C, to protect cytoplasm in cells, and fat-soluble antioxidants to protect the cell membranes, such as vitamin E. This is why using a combination of antioxidants is the most powerful approach.

Food antioxidants:

Wheatgrass juice
Freshly squeezed juices
   (drink quickly to prevent exposure to oxygen, which oxidises the antioxidants, rendering them ineffective)
Grapes (contains resveratrol)

Fun Fact: Resveratrol is a SIRT booster. SIRT is an anti-ageing enzyme. Grapes are your friend … and I don't mean wine! (You need to drink about 400ml of grape juice a day to increase your antioxidant status when the recommended daily amount is 150ml a day – this is equal to 1 glass.)

Reduce inflammation

The ageing process is sped up by chronic inflammation, which triggers free radicals that then activate the inflammatory cascade. The process ends with enzymes (Matrix metalloproteinases, aka MMPs[4]) breaking down your tissues, including collagen and elastin, which both give the appearance of plump skin.

The most common sources of chronic inflammation are:

UV radiation	Cosmetics or perfume
Heat	A diet with a high sugar content
Stress	Alcohol
Smoke pollution	Harsh weather

[Not so] Fun Fact: By your early thirties MMPs degrade collagen, and as you also produce less collagen, you should be getting your anti-ageing routine into full swing by then!

How to reduce and reverse the effects of chronic inflammation

The good news is that there are a few changes to your lifestyle that you can make that will help to reduce and reverse the effects of chronic inflammation, above and beyond a good anti-ageing skincare routine.

Anti-inflammatory ingredients for your diet to slow down ageing

Reduce your sugar! Sugar attaches to collagen (a process called 'glycation'), which makes it less elastic, while sugar also increases inflammation in the body.

Ginger, onions and garlic are all anti-inflammatory foods, so you may wish to incorporate these in your cooking.

Skincare ingredients that help boost collagen:

- Vitamins A, B, C, D and E
- Epigallocatechin Gallate (EGCG) from green tea
- Peptides
- Trace elements, including copper, iron, zinc and selenium

Reduce your stress levels

Tackling stress is important for so many reasons to support your wellbeing, but reducing your stress can also have a significant impact on your skin. *Stress ages you!*

Stress floods the body with cortisol and adrenaline, which raises blood sugar and insulin, which leads to inflammation, damaging the skin. Cortisol also reduces hyaluronic acid and leads to dry, dull skin.

Disrupted sleep can also cause cortisol to rise. The American Psychological Association have reported adults who **sleep fewer than eight hours a night** may have **higher stress levels** than those who sleep at least eight hours a night. Getting your beauty sleep is real!

Stress aggravates all existing skin conditions.

Whether it is acne, ageing or inflammation, it even takes longer for wounds to heal when you're stressed. Having a massage will stimulate oxytocin, which has a stress-buffering effect and reduces cortisol levels. Facial massage and face rolling can also be soothing for this reason.

Anti-ageing step-by-step routine

These anti-ageing ingredients should all be present in the skincare products you use:

Vitamins A, B, C and E

Green tea extract

Liquorice extract

Ferulic acid

Ergothioneine

The full skincare routine should include products that are ideally:

Fragrance free

Free of drying alcohols

Free of essential oils

Avoid harsh acids

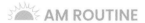 **AM ROUTINE**

Step 1: Begin with a micellar gel cleanse to wash away actives from the night before and any other dirt. Avoid soap and sodium lauryl sulphate.

Step 2: Moisturise with a fatty emollient and humectants, such as ceramides, peptides, urea and hyaluronic acid.

Step 3: Apply a physical SPF50 with zinc oxide to prevent any melasma, and antioxidants with a skin-neutral pH, such as vitamin E, green tea extract or resveratrol. This will help mop up any free radicals that develop during the day.

🌙 **PM ROUTINE**

Step 1: Double cleanse. Use an oil cleanser first to melt away makeup and sunscreen, then use a micellar gel wash to cleanse and hydrate the skin.

Step 2: Apply a light, hydrating, non-alcohol toner with humectants, soothers and brighteners, such as *Centella Asiatica*, allantoin, urea, panthenol and niacinamide.

Step 3: Use a gentle AHA exfoliator that includes mandelic or lactic acid. Avoid a product that includes over 5% glycolic as an exfoliator.

Step 4: Apply an antioxidant serum with vitamins A, C, E and green tea extract.

Step 5: Next, top off with a moisturiser that contains peptides and ceramides.

Step 6: Lastly, finish with a facial oil, such as squalene, marula oil, hemp seed oil or rose hip oil. Actives within the product should include tetrahexyldecyl ascorbate, retinaldehyde, retinol and retinyl palmitate, Coenzyme Q10, plus antioxidants.

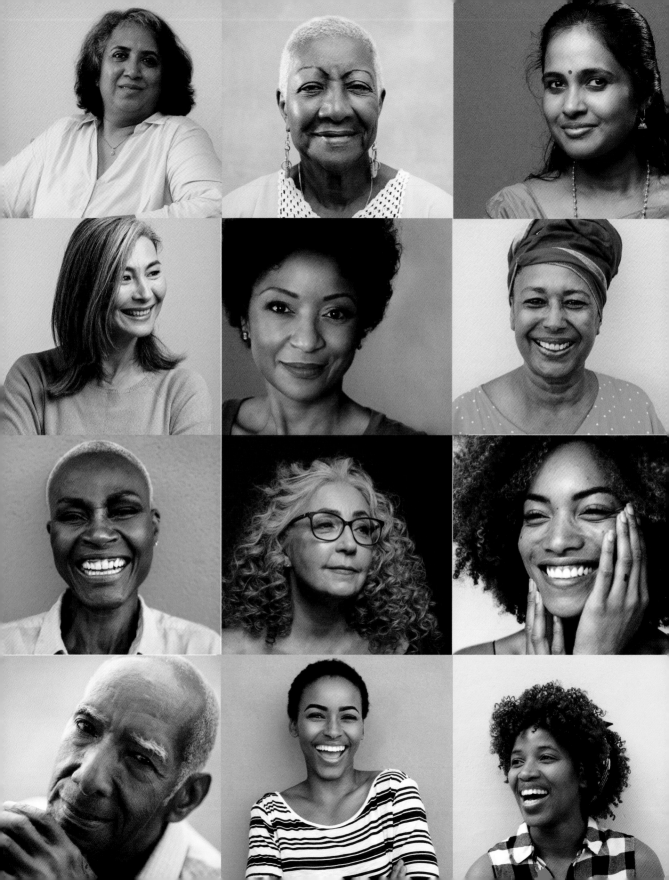

Skincare throughout the decades

This section will explain how your skincare routine will not remain the same forever, but will evolve throughout your lifetime as you and your skin ages. As every stage of your life presents different changes, I thought relaying this information as a breakdown by decade would be the most useful approach, and in each decade we will address the most common issues as well as how to create a routine that prevents premature ageing.

The skin is a huge organ, and with the following tips you can keep it in great shape even in old age. A youthful glow is for everybody – whatever your age!

My mum has been my reference point through the ages. She is absolutely stunning and has been blessed with great genes – she has never had a spot or even a dot of melasma. This meant she managed to get away with using just her moisturiser for decades. Now in her sixties, she is using chemical exfoliation, antioxidants and non-fragranced products and looks more than 10 years younger than her age. As you know, I inherit all the bad genes, so I have got started with this routine in my thirties!

Skincare in your twenties

Your skin at a cellular level

Early twenties

Collagen and elastin at its peak

Mid-twenties

Rate of collagen and elastin production decreases

Late-twenties

Hormone imbalance improves but may still break out

Ingredients to include ··········▶

Start using vitamin A, such as retinyl palmitate, retinol or retinaldehyde at night. Use SPF50 to slow ageing.

Use 0.5% salicylic acid wash or 2% salicylic acid toner. Use 2–5% benzoyl peroxide if needed.

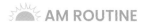 ## AM ROUTINE

Step 1: Cleanse to remove dirt, actives and dead skin cells.
Step 2: Use salicylic acid wash (if oily skin).
Step 3: Moisturise.
Step 4: SPF50 (reapply a couple of times during the day).

🌙 PM ROUTINE

Step 1: Double cleanse to remove makeup and sunscreen.
Step 2: If you have acne, use a salicylic acid wash (you can also use 2.5% benzoyl peroxide). For anti-ageing, include vitamin A (apply moisturiser first, then retinol, then moisturise again – this sandwich method will minimise irritation).
Step 3: Moisturise:
  If you have oily or acne-prone skin: apply gel and a light moisturiser.
  For anti-ageing: use a fatty, non-fragranced moisturiser, with vitamin A or other antioxidants.

My skincare confessions from my twenties

I would come back to halls of residence after a university night out and not bother to take off my makeup. I wasn't exactly subtle with my makeup either. For me, the blacker the eye liner the better, and I didn't know the meaning of choosing between heavy eyes or heavy lips! I was happy to go out with thick-rimmed dark eyes and my mum's bright red lipstick. All I can say is thank goodness it was before Facebook could record my inadequacy as a makeup artist!

Not only was my white pillow now black and blue from my eyeliner and eyeshadow, but my skin would break out and look dry and tired the next day. Terrible.

If I actually managed to take off my makeup before going to bed, I tugged at it with my supposedly hypoallergenic makeup wipes, not realising I still had plenty of gunk and grime left resting in my pores – yuck!

If you had asked me about SPF at that time I would have replied 'SP who?'. I thought this was only for hot, sunny holidays. I swiftly changed my mind later in my twenties when my mother pointed out the 'freckles' that had cropped up on my face were in fact the early signs of melasma!

The only reason I am willing to reveal all this and humiliate myself in such a public way is so that you and your children can do better than me!

Save your skin from your twenties – don't wait until your thirties or forties because then you are playing 'catch up'.

Skincare in your thirties

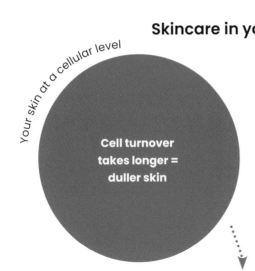

Your skin at a cellular level

Cell turnover takes longer = duller skin

Melanocytes start to be triggered, leading to tiny 'freckles'. This is early melasma and is a warning that you need to apply your SPF50 more vigilantly and reverse the melasma or it will spread

Ingredients to include ....▶

If you haven't started using vitamin A, start now. Exfoliate with lactic and mandelic acid to remove dull, dead skin.

Apply SPF50 every 2 hours.

No ingredients will reduce melasma if you haven't blocked the trigger.

Tyrosinase inhibitors, such as alpha arbutin, vitamin C, octadecenoic acid, liquorice extract, etc.

AM ROUTINE

Step 1: Cleanse (especially if you used vitamin A at night).
Step 2: Moisturise with a fatty, non-fragranced moisturiser (this separates the top layers of epidermis, which reduces the appearance of pigmentation and dull skin).
Step 3: Wear SPF50 and anti-melasma sunglasses and a SPF50 wide-brimmed hat.

🌙 PM ROUTINE

Step 1: Double cleanse to remove makeup and sunscreen.
Step 2: Apply toner with humectants as the first step to hydration.
Step 3: Exfoliate 1–2 times a week with a chemical exfoliant, so you are only removing dead skin cells.
Step 4: Apply tyrosinase inhibitors.
Step 5: Moisturise, as the second step to hydration.

My skincare confessions from my thirties

By this point, I had become pretty obsessive with applying my SPF50. I am a bit of an extremist, so it's all or nothing with me. Not only did I start walking around with SPF50 in my pocket, but even when sitting in a car I actually felt that the sun was glaring at my melasma, making it worse. So I attempted to look for anti-melasma sunglasses to cover my cheekbones (where my melasma lived). They didn't exist. I eventually went to an international sunglass-manufacturing fair in the hope of creating a pair of my own. You would think this should have been an easy thing to make, but it took two years to get a finished product. Most manufacturers looked at me like I was a little crazy when I explained how big I wanted my anti-melasma sunglasses to be. I finally achieved my goal with a boutique Italian workshop that made sunglasses by hand, one piece at a time.

When I first started wearing my Dr V sunglasses, I really didn't think anyone was as obsessed about their melasma as me, and I thought that the first batch I made would be my last, as only I'd want to wear them. It was only when my followers asked me about them and how to buy a pair that I realised I wasn't alone in my quest to keep my melasma at bay!

However, I was still eating like I was a student in my twenties well into my thirties. One of my many flaws is that I am a sugar addict. My high-sugar diet was encouraging inflammation and glycation, and I was also not using enough antioxidants in my skincare or consuming enough antioxidants in my diet. Thankfully I have managed to improve these habits by the time of writing this ... at 38 years of age!

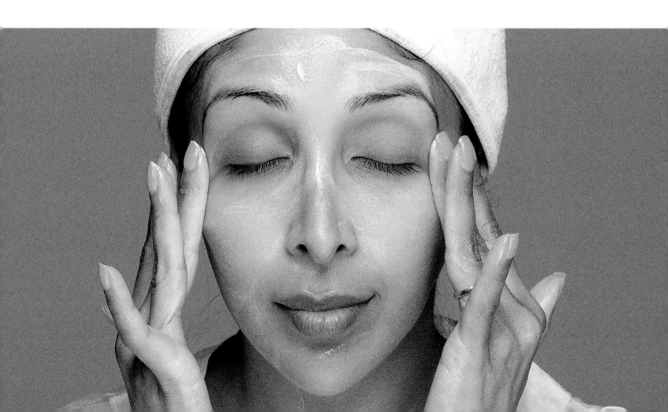

Dr V's Personal Skincare Routine in my thirties

(I am only including this because I get asked all the time what I do for my own skin – it is not intended for you to go and purchase these products.)

I have combination skin.

My main issues are melasma and ageing skin, I formulated and use the Dr Vanita Rattan range with these two concerns in mind.

AM ROUTINE

Step 1: Cleanse with Micellar Gel Wash.

Step 2: Apply Cera-Pep Brightening Moisturiser.

Step 3: Lastly, apply InZincable SPF50 (a mineral sunscreen with MelaShieldTM – this is a stem cell-vitamin complex we created to reduce hyperpigmentation during the day. It is UV stable and the independent clinical study on 51 skin of colour candidates showed 73% saw a reduction when switching from their regular SPF50 to Inzincable.)

PM ROUTINE

Step 1: Double cleanse with Oil Melting Cleanser and Micellar Gel Wash.

Step 2: Use a Super Hydrating Toner.

Step 3: Use the Exfoliate to Glow.

Step 4: Apply the Dr V Facial Pigmentation kit (for the cheekbones).

Step 5: Use the Anti-Oxidant Power Serum over the rest of the face.

Step 6: Lastly, apply Cera-Pep Moisturiser.

Skincare in your forties

In my forties I expect to go through menopause and the changes I expect will be drier skin, deeper wrinkles, larger pores, duller skin and more hyperpigmentation.

In anticipation of this, my routine will be tweaked to:

- Include more hydrating masks 2–3 nights a week. I would opt for cream masks as it is better for the environment.

- I will use my high-strength hyperpigmentation mask once a month to give an additional boost to the Dr V Facial Pigmentation kit for my melasma. Melasma is a chronic condition so it needs to be managed (see page 119).

- Habits I will need to enforce are sleeping on my back to reduce facial wrinkles, spending more time away from city pollution and eating more antioxidant foods, as well as increasing my protein and collagen intake. I should focus more on muscle work as opposed to cardio when I exercise, too, which has less impact on joints but will tighten loose body skin.

- From a cosmetic point of view, I will start to use lighter makeup, less powder and less heavy eye makeup.

Your skin at a cellular level

As oestrogen decreases, glycosaminoglycan decreases (water magnets). This means increased water evaporation from skin leading to dry skin

Loss of elastin causes a decrease in firmness and an increase in fine lines and loose skin, especially around eyes

Long-term UV exposure worsens any melasma, leading to fine lines

Ingredients to include

Need to add humectants, such as hyaluronic acid, urea, glycerine.

Need to trap water with occlusives such as petroleum, mineral oil, paraffin.

Strengthens skin barrier.

Stimulate collagen.

Vitamin A.

Fat-soluble vitamin C (tetrahexyldecyl ascorbate).

Peptides.

SPF50 on face and around eyes. Use anti-melasma sunglasses.

UPF50 wide-brimmed hat.

Tyrosinase inhibitors at night (see page 99).

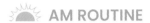 ## AM ROUTINE

Step 1: Cleanse, avoiding any harsh soaps or hot water.

Step 2: Moisturise with a fattier moisturiser and hyaluronic acid.

Step 3: Apply SPF50 every two hours, even on top of makeup, and UV daytime safe antioxidants.

PM ROUTINE

Step 1: Double cleanse, removing makeup and sunscreen.

Step 2: Tone with hyaluronic acid.

Step 3: Exfoliate two nights a week, avoiding harsh scrubs, and use chemical exfoliation such as mandelic or lactic acid to increase hydration.

Step 4: On non-exfoliating nights, moisturise, apply your retinol, then moisturise again. You can add a combination of fat-soluble vitamin C, peptides and tyrosinase inhibitors for anti-ageing and pigmentation. Moisturise with a fatty, non-fragrance moisturiser. Apply a barrier oil to triple hydrate and repair the skin barrier (such as toner, moisturiser and barrier oil).

Dr V's Top Tip:

In your forties your skin tends to be drier and not able to deal with environmental stress, such as pollution, as well as before. This is why hydration is key to create a healing environment for the skin. Fine lines around the eyes start to happen now, and the number one thing you must do is apply SPF50 around the eyes. This is an area that people may forget.

Classic skincare mistakes made in the forties

If you have never really been excited about skincare and you are trying to learn about it in your forties, it can be incredibly intimidating to know where to begin.

Don't waste your money on vitamin A (e.g. Retinol) if you aren't religiously applying your SPF50 every few hours. No skincare ingredient can beat UV on its own.

From various sources, you may take away that retinol is the main ingredient that you need for anti-ageing. However, this can lead to skin problems as retinol used at a high percentage (more than 0.5%) can lead to sensitivity and dry, flaking, dull skin.

You may think the sunscreen step doesn't feel that important as it's not really doing anything 'active' on your skin. This would be a mistake and may cause myriad problems.

Skincare in your fifties and beyond

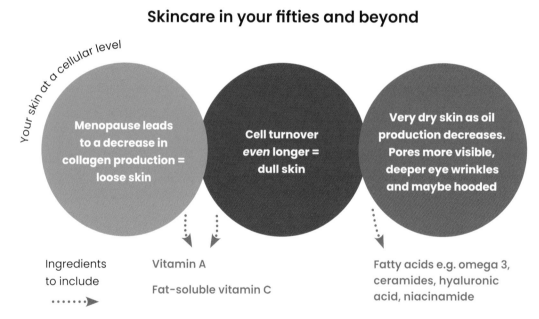

Your skin at a cellular level

Menopause leads to a decrease in collagen production = loose skin

Cell turnover *even* longer = dull skin

Very dry skin as oil production decreases. Pores more visible, deeper eye wrinkles and maybe hooded

Ingredients to include

Vitamin A

Fat-soluble vitamin C

Fatty acids e.g. omega 3, ceramides, hyaluronic acid, niacinamide

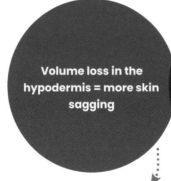

Volume loss in the hypodermis = more skin sagging

Inflammation means skin doesn't recover well from environmental stress, such as smoking, UV, pollution

Ingredients to include

Collagen procedures, such as fillers

Antioxidants and anti-inflammatory ingredients e.g. aloe, green tea

AM ROUTINE

Step 1: Cleanse with a micellar gel wash.
Step 2: Moisturise with a fatty moisturiser and hyaluronic acid.
Step 3: Apply SPF50 with antioxidants.

PM ROUTINE

Step 1: Double cleanse, removing makeup and sunscreen.
Step 2: Tone with niacinamide, hyaluronic acid and *Centella Asiatica*.
Step 3: Exfoliate with a hydrating chemical exfoliant, such as mandelic or lactic acid.
Step 4: Apply actives:
• Vitamin A – apply moisturiser first to decrease irritation.
• Fat-soluble vitamin C, vitamin E and Q10.
• Moisturise with a fatty, non-fragrance moisturiser, ceramides, peptides and barrier oil, such as marula or squalene.

Classic skincare mistakes made in the fifties and beyond

This is really when you see results of long SPF50 usage. It is easy to get lazy with SPF50 as you don't see immediate results from its application. It is usually decades later that we appreciate its importance.

If you are new to skincare at this point, go slow, as your skin won't tolerate a barrage of actives all at once.

The key here is to increase hydration first. This will immediately improve skin texture, brighten the skin and create a healing environment that is better equipped for environmental stress. Other gentle actives you can incorporate are:

- Tetrahexydecyl ascorbate – a skin brightener and antioxidant.
- Retinyl palmitate – to increase cell turnover and as an antioxidant.
- Tocopheryl acetate – anti-inflammatory and antioxidant.
- Green tea extract – anti-inflammatory.
- Aloe – anti-inflammatory.
- Ceramides – for skin barrier repair and as a moisturiser.
- Peptides – collagen stimulator and moisturiser.
- Hyaluronic acid – a water magnet.

Fun Fact: The MOST used skincare ingredient in the world is not what you might think!

... It is vitamin E (tocopheryl acetate).

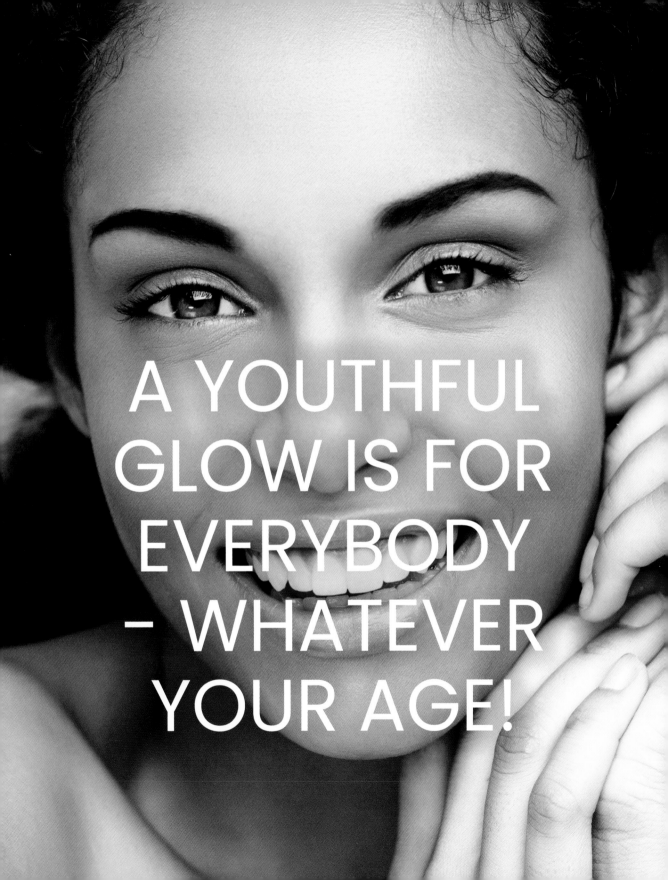

A YOUTHFUL GLOW IS FOR EVERYBODY – WHATEVER YOUR AGE!

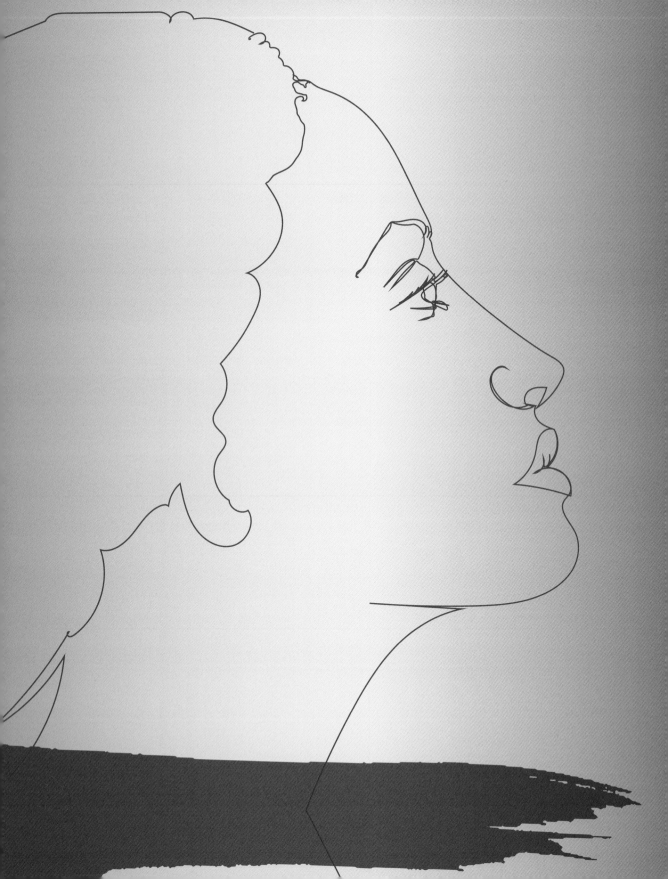

6

Attacking
ACNE

Acne is an incredibly common skin problem, affecting almost everyone at some stage of their life – 85% of young people between the ages of 12 and 24 years old and up to 35% of adults.

A chronic inflammatory condition seen as pimples, pustules or cysts on the skin, acne predominantly affects the face, chest and back – all the areas where there is a high density of hair follicles.

Acne can really crush your self-esteem, impact your wellbeing and contribute to depression and anxiety. It's often something that's more common in your teens, especially for men, when not only are your body and emotions changing rapidly, but you're also vying for the attention of your crush (if you're anything like me, although I repeatedly failed in my efforts!). The beauty standards of maintaining flawless skin just make the feeling of inadequacy worse. I hope this chapter holds your hand through this condition as I share the knowledge that I sorely wish I had had back then. One of the most important messages I am sharing with you here is that for acne, treatment should be sooner rather than later. While skincare can help treat acne, as I'll outline in the following sections, medical help from a dermatologist is highly recommended if you have a severe condition.

For me, acne has always been triggered by stress.

A study conducted on medical students between the ages of 22 and 24 years old showed a positive correlation between stress and acne severity[5]. By nature, I have always been a worrier; worrying about what may or may not happen has certainly aged my skin and at 38 years old I have now learnt to live in single-day compartments and simply enjoy the day that I find myself in without looking too far into the future. I have learnt to listen to my body and avoid known triggers.

Recently, I lived through a difficult time. I wasn't sleeping. I kept having heart palpitations. My hair was falling out, and when I looked in the mirror my face looked like it was under attack. I was used to getting the odd pimple the week before my period, and I didn't really suffer with acne as a teenager, but to have the huge stress I was under manifest itself on my face in horrific acne was a real eye-opener. My mum and dad asked me what happened, and how bad was it for my face to look like this? I'm sure they meant it in a loving way, but talk about hurting my self-esteem even more!

Acne is one of those things that you can see immediately on a person's face. Whether it's stress, financial issues, bereavement, illness or hormonal issues, acne is one of the ways these inner worries manifest on our skin. In an empowering Instagram post, actress Keke Palmer opened up about her issues with acne as a result of PCOS, and the emotional impact of it. I think it's important to have candid conversations about our skin and self-esteem, so that we can understand how these issues really affect us, and we can then learn how we can live better with them.

What I wish I could tell my younger self:

- Exercise daily – enjoy your body, it is a gift.

- Eat tons of vegetables and protein, your body will thank you.

- Stress is not worth it. You'll never think: 'I wish I had stressed more – life would have been so much better!'

- Meditate and detach yourself from negative stimuli around you. Be present in the moment. I ask myself a few times a day 'How are you feeling, Vanita? How is your heart feeling, how is your body feeling?' Then I take a big breath and say out loud how grateful I am for my life. I tell my husband and kids several times a day how grateful I am to have them in my life. I make gratitude my default emotion now, not the worry of what might happen or the fear that I'm not good enough.

Acne affects 80–90% of adolescents. Androgenic hormones (sex hormones) are considered one of the main causes of acne. (See pages 259–62 for pre-teen and teen skincare)

The 3 Ps are a guide to when hormonal acne is more likely to strike:

- Puberty
- Periods
- Pregnancy

What causes acne?

Acne is a complex condition, and there is no miracle cure for it. It is not as easy as 'cut dairy from your diet or stop using makeup' and your acne will go away. It occurs because of a complex interplay between a number of factors:

Hormones and bacteria – there is a surge in androgens (in particular the hormone testosterone) during puberty, which stimulates the growth of sebaceous glands, which in turn causes increased sebum production. This allows a bacteria – known as *Cutibacterium acnes* – which normally sits harmlessly on the skin, to colonise, and drive inflammation. As this is happening, a process called follicular hyperkeratinisation is taking place alongside this, where the cells lining the hair follicules become densely packed, causing the pores to become blocked. Blocked pores, excess oils and inflammation – a bad combination – are all drivers for acne.

Genetics – if there is a close family member who has or had acne, there is a higher risk of developing it yourself.

Other associated factors include:
- Cosmetics that cause skin trauma and are pore clogging (occlusion).
- Stress.

Where do your spots come from?

Normally, sebum is produced in the sebaceous gland from a duct that attaches to the hair follicle. Sebum rises to the surface to contribute to a healthy skin barrier and to lubricate the skin, keeping it hydrated.

In addition, skin cells that slough off in the hair follicle usually travel with the hair out of the pore just like a conveyor belt, running smoothly with no issues. This is why acne favours the upper trunks and face because there are lots of sebaceous glands here. The spots themselves that are produced go through different stages of development, starting with black heads and white heads.

What is the difference between a black head and a white head?

As spots begin to develop, first a plug is formed, which is a combination of sebum and dead skin cells in the hair follicle. If this plug is near the surface, the sebum oxidises (reacts with oxygen in the air) and it creates what is called a black head. If the plug is deeper in the follicle, then it is called a white head, because the air cannot reach the sebum and react with it to form a black head.

The white head can become more inflammatory and angry over time, presenting as small red bumps and pus-filled spots. It can also lead to deep red or dark painful large spots called nodules and cysts. This is a stage we do not want to get to, because this is where post-inflammatory hyperpigmentation and scarring happens, which is very difficult to treat.

Everyone's acne is unique.

While we all experience acne in different forms, to differing degrees of severity and extent, there are a few common things to look out for if you're not sure whether what you have is acne, a rash, or something else. Those are:

- Closed comedones (white heads).
- Open comedones (black heads).
- Papules or pustules (pus-filled spots).
- Nodules and cysts (painful inflamed areas of the skin).

The type of acne you have can also be influenced by your age. If you're a teenager, you will most likely have white heads and black heads on your forehead, nose and chin. If you're an adult, acne will crop up on your lower face and neck, and if you have periods you might experience PMS breakouts.

When it comes to skin of colour, we need to watch out for two common problems relating to acne:

Post-inflammatory hyperpigmentation (PIH)

Hyperpigmentation develops at the site of spots. Although PIH will resolve spontaneously, it can take weeks or months or even longer to fade without treatment. This is why we need to treat acne in skin of colour early.

Scarring

A common consequence of inflammatory acne (nodules and cysts). Although there are treatments such as microneedling, chemical peels and fillers that you can do, scarring can be even more challenging to treat than the acne itself. This is why we need to treat acne early, as scarring can be tricky to treat. I would advise to avoid spending money on any cosmetic products as the evidence behind their benefit in treating scars is weak. At this stage it would be valuable to see a dermatologist or cosmetic surgeon. Scarring is often one of the below types:

Atrophic – seen as ice pick, rolling and boxcar scars.

Hypertrophic – abnormal wound healing, there is an overproduction of tissue and the scar is raised.

Keloid scars – when scar tissue extends beyond the border of the original injury.

Acne is complex. There is no miracle cure for it. And it is not as easy to make disappear as life advice like 'cut dairy from your diet' or 'stop using make up' makes you believe.

Acne triggers and management

There are a few things you can do to prevent an outbreak.

- Use non-comedogenic makeup and creams to avoid clogging your pores.
- After exercise, wash the area. Avoid tight clothes that rub the back during exercise if you get back acne. Avoid backpacks as well.
- Avoid a high-glycaemic load diet for your general health and for your skin.

Acne can be treated with over-the-counter products that are not prescribed. However, if your acne continues to get worse, then it is important to see your doctor or get a referral to a dermatologist.

Acne-product ingredients

If you are buying products to treat your acne, there are some key ingredients you should look for in the packaging list.

Benzoyl peroxide 2.5% – this is best used for inflammatory and non-inflammatory acne. It 'poisons' the *Cutibacterium acnes* bacteria with oxygen, killing them off.

Benzoyl peroxide is also comedolytic, which means it exfoliates the skin and unclogs pores. However, it can take up 6 weeks to see results, and you might encounter side-effects such as flaking, sensitivity and dryness. This is why I recommend starting a couple of nights a week at 2.5% and only on the acne lesions, not everywhere. Be careful when applying it, as it can stain clothes. It can also increase the risk of sunburn, so using an appropriate sunscreen is recommended. I like to use a wash-off 5% BP, or Paula's Choice does a 2.5% cream.

Salicylic acid 2% – ideal for both white heads and black heads (non-inflammatory forms of acne), it is fat-soluble and penetrates the pore, and because it is a keratolytic, it dissolves the dead skin cells, unclogging the pores.

At 2% and less, salicylic acid acts as an anti-inflammatory and a keratolytic. At higher percentages it behaves as peeling agent, which is why I recommend a 2% leave-on product for acne.

Vitamin A – this is THE acne ingredient – remember, A for Acne! These are vitamin A-derived products that increase cell turnover and therefore unclog pores and stop black heads forming.

A slow and steady approach is important here. The aim is to build up tolerance to vitamin A so that it can be used daily, but at the beginning a twice-weekly application for a few weeks is recommended, with the aim of increasing use slowly over a few weeks or even months. It may take 2 to 3 cell cycles to see an improvement (about 8 to 12 weeks).

Use these products at night and remember to wear sunscreen during the day as retinol can be irritating.

A topical retinoid (vitamin A) and benzoyl peroxide are the treatment of choice, which you could incoporate into a routine by washing with benzoyl peroxide, then using vitamin A – such as The Ordinary 0.5% retinol or Paula's Choice 0.3% Retinol with Bakuchiol. Alternatively, you may be prescribed adapalene from a doctor.

You may see purging as pimples that are not yet visible come to the surface faster. This should subside within one cell cycle (4 to 6 weeks).

Oral retinoids (Isotretinoin) can be used for more severe cases of acne or acne that is not responding to topical treatments, if prescribed and safely monitored by a dermatologist.

Antibiotics – can be used as both topical creams or taken as a tablet prescribed by your doctor or dermatologist. The cream works against the acne-causing bacteria C. acnes, and it is often used in combination with benzoyl peroxide or a retinoid that helps fight the bacteria. The tablet has an anti-inflammatory effect and might be used if topical treatments are not working. The antibiotic family prescribed for acne would be tetracyclines – like doxycycline or lymecycline – which would normally be prescribed for no longer than three months.

Azelaic acid – this anti-bacterial, anti-inflammatory tyrosinase inhibitor helps with acne, PIE and PIH. The cosmetic formulations I recommend are 10% Azelaic acid booster from Paula's Choice, The Ordinary 10% Azelaic acid suspension or Naturium Azelaic Acid Emulsion 10%. This can also be prescribed at higher percentages (20%) by your GP or dermatologist.

Niacinamide 2–5% – this isn't generally used as first-line treatment in acne, but it may help where other recommended products are not tolerated.

Niacinamide will improve sebum control and helps brighten the skin, which is useful with PIH.

Hormonal treatments – the combined oral contraceptive pill has a role in treating acne in women who require contraception. They work by reducing sebum production and androgen levels.

Spot treatments – spot treatments are not a substitute for acne treatment – which requires treatment of the whole area. However, treating individual spots can be useful sometimes (hello, mega zit that appeared out of nowhere at the most inconvenient time!). The routine overleaf is my go-to in these cases, and aims to lift pus and oil and reduce pimple size.

ACNE skincare plan

If you suffer from acne, try this daily skincare routine. Also, if you break out the week before your period you can switch to this routine to minimise acne.

- Benzoyl peroxide
- Retinoid

- Salicylic acid
- Hydrocolloid patches

 ## AM ROUTINE

Step 1: Cleanse with Inky List salicylic acid.
Step 2: Apply niacinamide The Ordinary.
Step 3: Use a non-comedogenic moisturiser, such as Super Gel from Face Theory.
Step 4: SPF50 Cerave Mineral (it does look white on skin, though).

 ## PM ROUTINE

Step 1: Cleanse with 5% benzoyl peroxide Acnecide.
Step 2: Use a vitamin A, such as 0.5% Retinol from The Ordinary.
Step 3: Apply a non-comedogenic moisturiser, such as Super Gel from Face Theory.

Common mistakes:

Scrubbing skin to try to remove the oil 'slick'. This is inflamed skin, so scrubbing the skin can cause micro tears.

Starting your skincare routine late or once acne has developed. I recommend a basic oil-controlling routine from 11 years old if the skin looks congested. (See pages 259–62 for pre-teen and teen acne advice.)

Using alcohol toners to try to remove the oil. This gives temporary satisfaction, but the acne will come back faster and often worse as the feedback loop is that the skin feels dry.

DIY skincare from watching social media videos, for example, using toothpaste on acne breakouts. This is an irritant, why do this to already inflamed skin?

Using pore-clogging makeup to hide acne can make the situation worse. It is better to stick with a colour corrector just on the PIH and brown marks and maybe a powder for the rest of the face. Try to keep it minimal.

Not cleansing the face properly (using makeup wipes doesn't count). Grime, creams and dirt are stuck in the pores, contributing to breakouts.

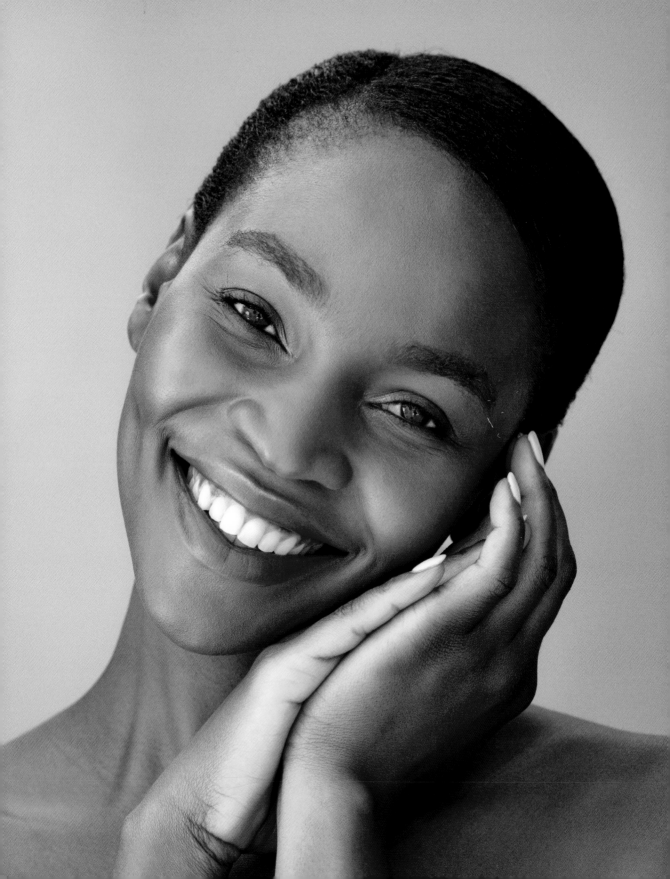

Acne and bacteria

1. Increased androgen hormones, such as dihydrotestosterone, will increase sebum production.

2. Increased sebum production will trigger hyperkeratosis, the production of excess keratin. Keratin is a protein that makes dead skin cells stick together and unable to leave the hair follicle as usual. This forms a plug, blocking the sebaceous duct leading out of the pore.

3. There is now an oxygen-deprived (anaerobic) area, and guess which bacteria loves its anaerobic environment? Yes, C. acnes (formerly known as Propionibaterium acnes acnes).

C. acnes is thought to colonise the skin in children between 11 and 15 years old, which is why we start seeing acne at this time. I recommend starting a skincare routine from 11 years old, especially for our skin-of-colour children, because controlling acne early will reduce acne scars and pigmentation later.

What does C. acnes do?

C. acnes triggers more free fatty acids in your skin, leading to inflammation and possible hyperpigmentation and/or scars and ultimately, harder to treat acne. Here's the science behind it:

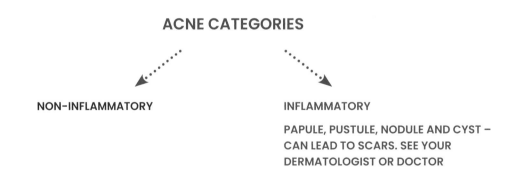

ACNE CATEGORIES

NON-INFLAMMATORY

INFLAMMATORY

PAPULE, PUSTULE, NODULE AND CYST – CAN LEAD TO SCARS. SEE YOUR DERMATOLOGIST OR DOCTOR

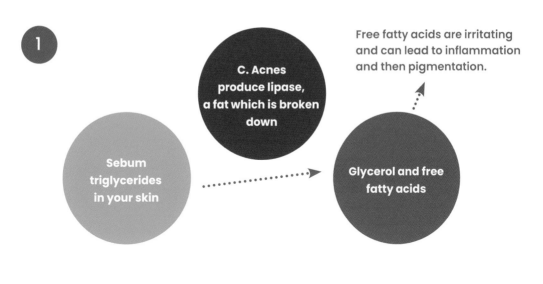

1

C. Acnes produce lipase, a fat which is broken down

Sebum triglycerides in your skin

Glycerol and free fatty acids

Free fatty acids are irritating and can lead to inflammation and then pigmentation.

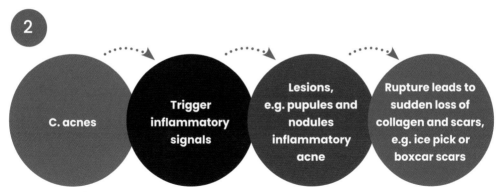

2

C. acnes

Trigger inflammatory signals

Lesions, e.g. pupules and nodules inflammatory acne

Rupture leads to sudden loss of collagen and scars, e.g. ice pick or boxcar scars

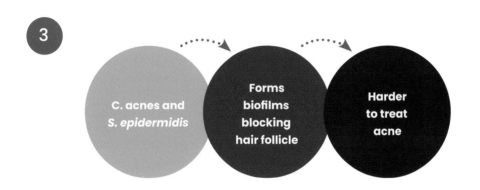

3

C. acnes and *S. epidermidis*

Forms biofilms blocking hair follicle

Harder to treat acne

MYTH: Acne is due to poor skin hygiene.

TRUTH: The plug forms in the new hair follicle, not on the skin surface, so how can it be due to hygiene? We all have C. acnes on our skin. This is also not a hygiene issue. In fact, over-washing will lead to further irritation of already inflamed skin.

MYTH: Acne is contagious.

TRUTH: We all already have this bacteria on our skin. Acne develops when the correct environment exists for C. acnes to replicate.

MYTH: Squeezing the spot is the quickest way to get rid of a spot.

TRUTH: Unfortunately doing this damages the already weak and inflamed pore. This is why you tend to get recurring acne in the exact same location. A steroid (cortisone) injection by your dermatologist will reduce a spot if you have an important event coming up. This is not a 'normal' measure, though, it is the exception.

Sudden acne in adult women

If you also experience irregular periods and excess hair growth (on the face and body), it could be due to a hormonal imbalance called polycystic ovary syndrome. Your doctor can usually diagnose it using an ultrasound and blood test.

How acne skincare ingredients work

Firstly, you should only use over-the-counter creams for mild or moderate acne. If it is painful, inflamed with cysts, then you must see your dermatologist. For skin of colour, inflammation is bad news as it leads to hyperpigmentation. This can take months or years to get rid of (please read the tyrosinase inhibitors chapter on page 99). In addition, the cysts can burst, which leads to a sudden loss of collagen, which in turn leads to scarring and uneven skin texture.

Thinking holistically about skin

If I had followed the below advice from my future self, I would probably have been a happier soul and had more beautiful skin, but my younger self would probably not have listened. How many times have we ignored our own parents' advice? It is only when we see the results of our actions that we change our habits. I am waiting for the day that my daughter Sienna ignores my advice!

In terms of habits I'm proud to have developed, a daily skincare routine is one. It is a small thing I can do every day that doesn't take long, but it gives me the satisfaction of knowing I am taking good care of myself. And this in turn means that my self-esteem is boosted and I continue to practise kindness towards myself – healing my skin when it's inflamed or hurting.

I know it seems so easy for me to say, 'Just destress your life'. Of course, I know life isn't quite as easy as that. Our amygdala (the structure in the brain that processes emotion) is very good at putting us into fight or flight mode, which helped our ancestors survive but for modern-day life it is not so helpful and chronic stress affects all organs of our body. I want better for you and for our children.

Red acne vs brown acne marks

As I age, it takes longer and longer for the cycle to create new skin cells. So it takes longer and longer for my skin to recover from post-inflammatory erythema and post-inflammatory hyperpigmentation. This is when you start taking your skin more seriously!

When I go through a bout of stress, my skin erupts with spots. This is exacerbated by my monthly couple of spots the week before my period. It will then take me about 12 weeks (2–3 cell cycles) to clear my skin of the pigmentation (brown marks).

Post-inflammatory Erythema (PIE) are the red, burgundy or deep purple marks left after inflammation caused by damage to capillaries (blood vessels) that are close to the skin's surface.

In skin of colour:

- Post-inflammatory Erythema (PIE) can become red, burgundy or brown marks (PIH).
- Post-inflammatory Hyperpigmentation (PIH) is when your melanocytes (melanin-producing cells) produce increased pigment, which is seen on the surface as hyperpigmentation.

Important to note:

The treatment of PIE and PIH is different as PIE is not a pigmentation problem.

Why acne can lead to longer-term issues in skin of colour:

- For skin of colour, acne is a triple threat.
- We get the acne, the red mark and then the brown marks.
- Often the red and brown marks are more psychologically painful than the original spot.

Which do you scar more with, red or burgundy marks or brown marks?

Red marks (PIE) (779 responses) **Brown marks (PIH)** (2609 responses)

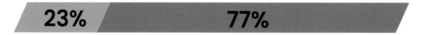

23%   77%

How can you tell if it is PIE or PIH?

Sometimes the red marks start to become darker but you are not sure if it is still PIE or now PIH.

Quick test:

Use a glass and press it up to your skin.

- If the marks disappear, it is PIE, this is because PIE is a blood vessel, which will disappear on compression.
- If it is PIH, the marks stay, because pigmentation of the skin isn't affected by blood supply.

Key actives for PIE

Salicylic acid	Helps to decrease acne by unclogging pores and is anti-inflammatory
Azelaic acid	Anti-inflammatory and antibacterial
Niacinamide	Reduces erythema
Vitamin C (not ascorbic acid)	Powerful antioxidant – it prevents free radicals from causing further inflammation
Green tea extract	Anti-inflammatory and antioxidant
Aloe, panthenol, bisabolol	Skin soothers
Hyaluronic acid, ceramides, NMF	Protects skin barriers and acid mantle of skin Hydration is essential to repair the skin
SPF50	Avoid UV causing free radicals, leading to further inflammation

Key actives for PIH

Niacinamide	**Melanosome transfer interrupter**
Retinoids	**Tyrosinase inhibitor**
Alpha arbutin	**Tyrosinase inhibitor**
Kojic dipalmitate	**Tyrosinase inhibitor**
Vitamin C (e.g. ascorbyl phosphate and tetrahexyldecyl ascorbate)	**Tyrosinase inhibitor**
Vitamin E (tocopheryl acetate)	**Tyrosinase inhibitor**
Green tea extract	**Tyrosinase inhibitor**
Liquorice extract	**Tyrosinase inhibitor**
Hyaluronic acid	**Moisturise (humectant)**
Glycerine	**Moisturise (humectant)**
Broad spectrum (e.g. zinc oxide or tinosorb M)	**SPF50**

What do you do if you have both PIE and PIH?

I recommend the following actives:

Salicylic acid	unclogs pores
Niacinamide	controls sebum production
Retinoids	increases cell turnover and antioxidant
Vitamin C (e.g. sodium ascorbyl phosphate and tetrahexyldecyl ascorbate), green tea extract	tyrosinase inhibitor and antioxidant
Alpha arbutin, kojic dipalmitate, liquorice extract	tyrosinase inhibitor
Hyaluronic acid, glycerine	humectant i.e. water magnet
Broad spectrum SPF50 sunscreen, e.g. zinc oxide	anti-inflammatory

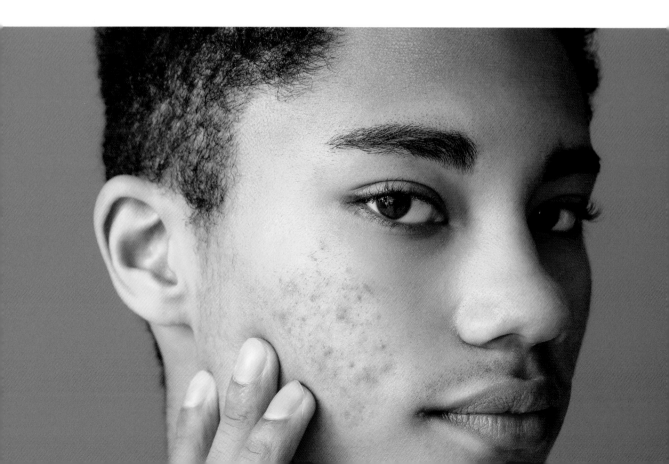

Dr V's Formulation Insights

This is the process I go through to create a product to address an issue.

Firstly, I figure out which percentages are needed and how they can be combined at their optimal pH levels. Often this isn't possible and you may need a kit of two or even three products to ensure you get every ingredient you can at the correct percentage.

This is what I did with the facial pigmentation kit to address PIE and PIH.

It is also important to follow up with a clinical study to see if your theory holds up. This is not a legally required step and is at the discretion of the manufacturing company – and it is an expensive step. This is how manufacturers are able to create products that don't match up to the claims, as no proof is required.

You, however, will not be duped as you know exactly what you are looking for on packaging!

The landscape has become dominated by single actives. The Ordinary started a skincare revolution, which democratised skincare. They suddenly allowed the majority to purchase good-quality actives in the therapeutic range. They then inspired a large number of companies to follow this, as the model was so popular.

The downside is when you are dealing with multiple pathologies, single actives just aren't good enough. The reason being, once you layer the third single-ingredient serum onto the skin you are not getting much penetration, so there is minimal efficacy.

This is why I prefer formulating cocktail creams with between 10–15 actives to deal with multi-pathology conditions.

Cystic acne

When pores become swollen with sebum, bacteria and dead skin cells it can cause
a cyst. The cyst is deeper in the skin and can be painful. If a cyst bursts it can lead to
textured scarring (atrophic scarring). Over-the-counter products are unlikely to work for
cystic acne, so please visit your dermatologist. Waiting can mean the scar is permanent
and this can be traumatic. A dermatologist will most likely prescribe you Roaccutane.
Cystic acne must be dealt with quickly and professionally.

Hypopigmentation

One in twenty people have at least one hypopigmented patch of skin on their body. It is
far more obvious in skin of colour, though, which can lead to panic.

The most common causes are:

- **Pityriasis versicolor** – a very common yeast infection on the face and trunk of
  the body, especially in children. It may resolve itself or you can use ketoconazole
  shampoo on the hypopigmented patches.
- **Post-Inflammatory Hypopigmentation** – this is one reason why I don't
  recommend hyperpigmentation treatments that are too harsh for the skin, such
  as hydroquinone, which can cause PIH as a side effect.
- **Vitiligo** – this is an auto-immune condition where there is death of the melanocyte.
  It often starts before 30 years of age and may spread with time. There have been
  promising results with UV light therapy and mesenchymal stem cell therapy.
- **Pityriasis alba** – very common, affecting 5% of children worldwide. It usually
  resolves within 1 year. If it is itchy you can use a low-dose steroid cream,
  e.g. 0.5% hydrocortisone. If it is dry, use a thick moisturiser.
- **Halo naevin** – a hypopigmented halo ring around the mole that is thought to be
  auto-immune.

Back acne

I bet you didn't know that your back has almost as many oil-producing glands as your face? Excess dead skin cells clumping with excess oil inside your back's pores will block them, causing inflammation and triggering the much-maligned bacne.

Any activity that causes sweating, friction and irritation on the back creates the perfect environment for back acne. Playing lots of sports where you sweat and wear tight-fitting clothing, or even the friction from a backpack can be enough to trigger a flare up.

In the Hyperpigmentation Clinic, I often saw men in their mid-20s to mid-50s wanting to treat post acne pigmentation on the upper and lower back, whereas women would more commonly ask for help with upper-back acne. Back acne can stop people from wearing certain clothes for fear of revealing their skin.

Some people use foundation to cover up back acne, but this tends to come off on clothes, which feels like an additional restriction.

Often back acne spreads to the shoulders and buttocks. Please read the beginning of this chapter to fully understand what is actually happening in the skin during an acne breakout (see page 168).

To treat back acne you need to:

- Eliminate excess sebum
- Unclog pores
- Kill C. acnes bacteria
- Prevent skin inflammation

To achieve the above, the ingredients you need are:

- Anti-inflammatory
- Antibacterial
- Moisturising
- Will absorb excess oil

Choose a body wash with the following ingredients:

1. Salicylic acid – a BHA which unblocks the pores of sebum and dead skin.

2. Mandelic acid or lactic acid – AHAs that dissolve the upper layer of the skin to prevent spots and help with hyperpigmentation.

Step-by-step routine for back acne

- Wash the area with a 5% benzoyl peroxide product. A benzoyl peroxide wash will kill the bacteria and break up lesions. Use it consistently, leave it on the skin for 2–5 minutes and then wash off so it doesn't stain clothes (unlike creams) – 5% is effective and less irritating than 10%.

- If there is no sensitivity you can use a 2% salicylic acid, leave-on exfoliant to unclog pores.

- Apply a vitamin A cream daily, such as Differin. Apply to moisturised skin after a shower if you find it too irritating. Use a back applicator for hard-to-reach areas.

- Fabric softeners, bars of soap (solidifying additives can cause problems) and hard water can affect the composition of oil and lead to clogging of pores.

Don't re-use towels, and wash sheets and pillows regularly, as bacteria builds up

Lifestyle changes

There are a few changes you can make to day-to-day living that will help to improve the condition:

- Wear loose-fitting clothes, especially when working out.
- Avoid friction on affected areas, such as from backpacks.
- Shower straight after going to the gym or any activity where you have sweated a lot. If this is not possible, use salicylic wipes to remove sweat and avoid picking or squeezing spots!
- You may also want to use a salicylic acid spray as a 'post-workout acne' treatment and change clothes.
- Avoid harsh or sensitising products that include denatured alcohol, essential oils or fragrance.
- Wear your non-comedogenic SPF50 when the back is exposed or pigmentation may develop.

Common mistakes:

Never scrub acne in the shower as it aggravates the skin barrier. More TEWL leads to inflammation, which can trigger a flare up.

Malassezia folliculitis – also known as fungal acne

'I have a sudden crop of itchy bumps on my face.'

Malassezia is a yeast that lives naturally on the skin. However, an overgrowth can cause an infection in the hair follicles and looks like tiny, uniform (exactly the same size), itchy spots. These spots will appear on your forehead, temples and frontal hair line – but the upper chest, back and shoulders can be affected, too. While Malassezia infection can seem like a regular breakout, it does not respond to typical treatments for acne – which can leave you frustrated if you don't know what you're dealing with.

Is it fungal acne or bacterial acne?

Fungal acne is:

Itchy
Uniform in size and colour
Clustered together

Unlike bacterial acne, which is:

Not itchy
Different sizes with PIE and PIH
(red marks and brown marks)
Spread out randomly

Causes and triggers

There are several causes and triggers for fungal acne, and sometimes a few lifestyle changes can be made to help to avoid breakouts.

• Fungal acne loves a warm, humid environment – avoid wearing tight-fitting clothing.
• Personal hygiene – sweating will create the perfect environment, so shower after the gym, wash the face during the day and wash clothes between workouts.
• Don't wear a heavy layer of creams or makeup that blocks hair follicles.
• Antibiotics or immune-suppressing drugs can trigger this, so be aware of any signs so you can take prompt preventative action.

Treatment

Try these options to see which has the best effect on your acne. Start with shampoo, as this is cheap and easy to obtain, then upgrade to a leave-on cream.

- Anti-fungal 2% ketoconazole shampoo. Leave on for 3–5 minutes and rinse off. Use 3–4 times a week during a breakout. Continue once a week for three months to avoid relapse.
- Other over-the-counter treatments: topical fungal creams – miconazole/ clotrimazole – usually apply once or twice daily. Sometimes anti-fungal tablets are needed.
- Use 2% BHA leave-on exfoliant to unclog pores. Follow with a non-comedogenic moisturiser.

Malassezia is nourished by oil – either sebum or oil formula creams – this is why it affects oil-rich areas of the face, including the forehead, nose and chin. It takes weeks or even months to see an improvement. If this fails, then it is important to see your doctor or get a referral to a dermatologist.

Additional steps:

- Avoid using oils on the face and avoid using makeup and hair oil until the acne resolves.
- Assess your lifestyle – stress can exacerbate any skin condition, including fungal acne.
- There is a tendency for fungal acne to come back, so maintenance treatment may be needed.

Hormonal acne (monthly period-related acne)

My husband is more tuned into my 'time of the month' than I am. I have a 'signalling' phrase I say once a month the day before my period.

'I feel so sad and I don't know why.'

My husband hugs me and says, 'Your skin is also breaking out.'

We both laugh because we know what is about to happen. My seven-year-old daughter even knows!

I thought it was just me that went through this, it is not something we discuss publicly but the older I got the less I felt I needed to hide 'embarrassing' things, the more I talked to my friends and realised this affected every woman that I knew.

What follows are my findings from an Instagram poll I conducted on this subject.

How many of you experience monthly hormonal acne?

Yes (3,327 responses) **No** (542 responses)

86%	14%

How many of you experience acne in the week leading up to your period?

1 week before (2,541 responses) **During period** (803 responses)

76%	24%

Dr V's Interpretation: monthly hormonal acne is incredibly common and tends to occur one week before your period. Considering this is the case, it surprises me that we don't discuss women having a cyclical skincare routine.

I write in my diary when my period is and I switch from my melasma, anti-ageing routine to my hormonal acne routine one week before I am due to start my period.

Why does this happen?

HORMONAL ACNE

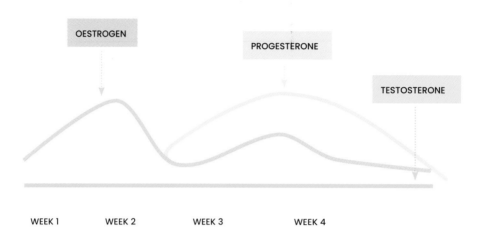

In the Luteal phase, days 14–23, progesterone rises, which stimulates sebum production and mild acne.

First half of period cycle

- This is when the oestrogen level is relatively high.
- Oestrogen is important because it improves the skin barrier, supports collagen production and improves hydration and wound healing.

It is suggested that the reduction of oestrogen during menstruation (your period) is the reason for sensitive skin. You may also note that waxing or threading at this time is particularly painful, I know I do!

> I incorporate a salicylic acid mask the week before my period and use a BHA 2% toner every night to minimise the chances of getting a spot.

Second half of the cycle

Progesterone at this time stimulates sebum production and the pores minimise, trapping sebum. This is the luteal phase and mild acne can develop.

> Start using 2% salicylic acid mask followed by niacinamide.

Menstruation

When you start your period, there is a relatively higher testosterone level, which is thought to further stimulate sebum production, which in turn can cause a breakout.

Apply 2.5% benzoyl peroxide directly onto the spot.

Do you feel sad before your period?

Low mood and irritability may occur during a specific time frame called the luteal phase. This usually happens in the last week of your cycle before menstruation, which is why it coincides with acne breakouts.

Yes (2,626 responses)   **No** (698 responses)

| 79% | 21% |

You are NOT alone, I am right there with you.

The good news is that both mood and skin immediately improve after menstruation. It is important to remember that stress can exaggerate all skin conditions, including acne, so this is another key time to practise self-care!

I usually switch to my oily acne routine one week before I'm due my period – I avoid oil cleansers, use salicylic acid exfoliant from Paula's Choice and a non-comedogenic gel moisturiser from Face Theory and I am ready with my pimple patches, e.g. 'dots for spots'.

Suggested oily acne routine:

 AM ROUTINE

Step 1: Salicylic acid wash
Step 2: Niacinamide serum
Step 3: Non-comedogenic moisturiser
Step 4: SPF50

☾ **PM ROUTINE**

Step 1: Micellar gel wash
Step 2: Benzoyl peroxide on spots (wait until it dries so doesn't make retinol ineffective)
Step 3: 0.5% retinol serum
Step 4: Non-comedogenic moisturiser

Dehydrated skin with acne

This is one of the most frustrating skin combinations, as the majority of products for acne contain higher percentages of benzoyl peroxide, salicylic acid and vitamin A, which are excellent ingredients but can dry the skin. When overused or no moisturiser is applied on top it can lead to dry skin.

First you need to figure out if you have **dry skin** or **dehydrated skin**. These are two different issues with different causes and solutions.

Dehydrated skin is a condition characterised by lack of water in the top layer of skin. The skin may be oily simultaneously, so the skin can feel dry, look oily and get spots all at the same time.

Dry skin is a skin type characterised by not enough skin fats, which means water evaporates faster from the surface. The skin barrier is chronically compromised but doesn't usually breakout.

Dehydrated skin feels:

- Dry
- Sensitive
- Dull
- Rough
- Shows rapid fine lines and sagging

The most common cause of acne on dry skin is *damage to the skin barrier* **with sensitising or irritating skin products and practices, such as:**

- Over-scrubbing or over-exfoliation
- Overuse of benzoyl peroxide, vitamin A or salicylic acid
- Fragrance
- Essential oils
- Denatured alcohol

External factors can also play a part in dehydrating skin, for example:

- Weather, especially UVA rays
- Pollution
- Hormones
- Hard water from showers (please avoid hot showers and baths – ensure water is lukewarm; you can use a water softener, too)
- With ageing we lose ceramides in the skin
- Air-conditioning and central heating further dehydrate the skin

How to treat dehydrated acne skin

The aim is to replenish the skin and hydrate it.

First you need to use water magnets (humectants) to hold water in the epidermis. Use fats as emollients to smooth skin cells and repair the barrier. I would recommend using the below anti-inflammatory ingredients to soothe dehydrated, irritated skin.

- Fatty acids
- Cholesterol
- Ceramides
- Hyaluronic acid

- Glycerine
- Urea
- Panthenol
- Aloe

Routine

Your daily routine needs to start with hydrating the skin before applying any actives, to reduce any chances of irritation.

- Hydrating cleanser
- Hydrating toner
- Use 2% BHA with humectants on the acne breakouts

  Hopefully no other actives are needed and you can go straight to moisturising but if not you need benzoyl peroxide 2.5% max as it is very drying. It kills the C. acnes *bacteria. Only use it on the acne lesion, not the whole face.)*

- You then need to hydrate again – use a non-comedogenic moisturiser
- During the day wear sunscreen. I like zinc oxide, which is an anti-inflammatory and antimicrobial (mineral sunscreen)

When you wash your face, please don't put it under a hot shower!

Always use lukewarm water; hot water is so bad for our skin, especially dry skin.

Dry skin

With dry skin the barrier function is impaired. There may be fewer 'fats' that retain water in the skin, such as ceramides, cholesterol and free fatty acids. This is why it is usually called 'dehydrated acne skin' not 'dry acne skin'.

You need to avoid all irritants and be gentle with the skin. (I recommend you read the eczema chapter for a step-by-step routine.)

The first thing you need to do is repair the skin barrier with emollients and humectants.

The symptoms of a damaged skin barrier include:

- Erythema (redness or a burgundy colour)
- Dry, itchy, flaky skin
- Skin sensitivity
- Skin looking dull, dry, rough but also oily

Causes of a damaged skin barrier

- The most common cause of a damaged skin barrier is over-washing. This decreases fats on the skin, which is the first barrier to skin irritants.
- Over-exfoliation does the same thing. I recommend avoiding physical or enzyme exfoliants.
- Environmental assaults, including dry central heating or air conditioning, cold weather, wind and pollution – all of these damage our skin barrier. We all need strong humectants, antioxidants and SPF50 in our basic skincare routine.
- The skin barrier is weakened with age as there is a decrease in skin ceramides.

How to repair your skin barrier

My skin barrier has been damaged three times in my lifetime, and on each occasion it was because I didn't take my own advice and instead followed skincare trends without understanding the science behind them – a BAD idea!

The first time, I was trying to treat my melasma in my late twenties and I over-exfoliated with a well-known face scrub. I noticed how 'bright' my skin looked the next day, but after the third harsh scrub that week I noticed my skin felt very sensitive and it stung with my normal melasma actives – even starting to flake. I could see red patches developing on the tops of my cheeks. This had never happened to me before.

The second time it happened to me was when I was gifted a well-known 1% retinol serum and after two nights' use (not consecutive) my skin felt tender and flaked.

The third time was when I decided to try a natural deodorant. Please read the underarm hyperpigmentation section (see page 138) to learn what happened with that one!

Every time after these actions I was forced to stop my skincare routine and allow my skin to repair itself.

Prevention is key here; if you are prone to sensitive, dry skin or chronic inflammation, avoid known irritants or skin sensitisers in your skincare and makeup, including fragrance, denatured alcohol and essential oils. If the skin is damaged it allows increased TEWL (water evaporation) and more irritants to enter, which increases inflammation and causes further damage.

Once your skin barrier has been damaged

If the damage has been done, simplify your skincare routine. Quickly wash your face with lukewarm water and only use a mild cleanser *that does not have* sodium lauryl sulfate. Use a broad-spectrum mineral sunscreen to minimise any irritation during the day – zinc is good as it reduces inflammation.

Some other ingredients to avoid are:

- Alkaline soaps or stripping agents, such as denatured alcohol.
- Don't use physical harsh scrubs or scrubbing tools, which can lead to micro tears.
- Actives that irritate the skin if you are prone to skin burning, as this exacerbates damage.
- Alpha hydroxy acids such as glycolic, lactic or mandelic acids, BHAs (drying), such as salicylic acid.
- Vitamin A.

Key actives you need in your skincare

(not all but the majority ideally)

To replace fatty acids	ceramides peptides
Humectants	hyaluronic acid urea glycerine
Occlusives and emollients	paraffinum liquidum petrolatum
Anti-inflammatory	green tea extract aloe panthenol
Additional barrier oil (PM use only)	marula oil squalane

Ingredients I love for dry skin with acne:

Petrolatum	Hyaluronic acid
Mineral oil	Glycerine
Ceramides	Silicone, such as
Peptides	cyclopentasiloxane

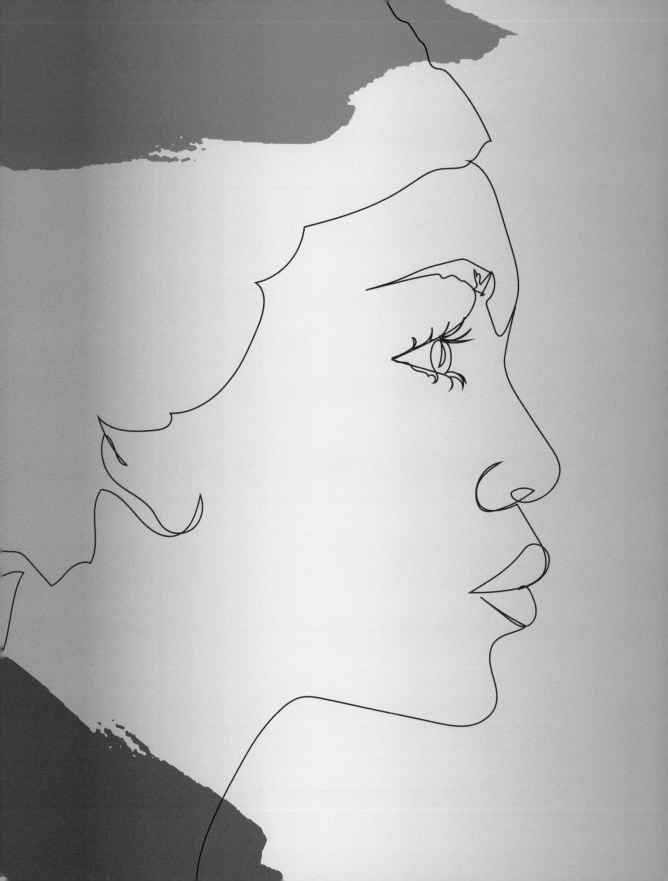

7

ECZEMA

Eczema is a chronic, itchy, inflammatory skin condition. You most likely know someone who is affected by it, as it's extremely common. It affects all age groups but most frequently occurs in childhood, in up to one in five children.

My son was prone to eczema and as a parent I know it's easy to worry you have done something to cause it – used the wrong detergent or product, for instance – but the truth is eczema is multifactorial. There is no known single cause, but risk factors are genetic and environmental – all can lead to problems with your skin barrier. This includes:

- Water loss from the skin, leading to dryness and itching.
- It makes the skin more susceptible to allergens and irritants.
- It predisposes the skin to infection from *Staphylococcus aureus* (presents as redness, oozing and crusting of the skin).

Eczema can be very difficult to live with, affecting many different areas of your life, from your self-confidence, your sleep (and in turn your ability to work or go to school), to your social life and mental health.

Another term for eczema is atopic dermatitis. Eczema is extremely common and a clear sign is itching, which can sometimes be intense enough to keep you up at night, scratching away.

Other symptoms include:

- Redness or burgundy colour of inflamed areas
- Uncomfortable feeling, dry skin
- Thickening of skin lines (lichenification)

Chronic scratching can tear the skin, which leaves your skin vulnerable to infections. It also thickens the skin and can lead to hyperpigmentation.

In darker, pigmented skin eczema appears ashen, greyish in colour rather than red and you can develop small bumps surrounding your hairs. Lichenification (see below) is more common in darker pigmented skin, and dryness of the skin tends to be more extensive – you'll also be more likely to get dry circles of skin surrounding your eyes. You can develop hyper- or hypopigmentation if you scratch too much.

Eczema goes through several stages of severity as your skin barrier becomes more and more compromised. Secondary infection from bacteria, such as staphylococcal and streptococcal bacteria, can also occur when the skin barrier function is impaired.

Acute stage

Seen as swollen greyish or red patches; there may be oozing, crusting and small fluid-filled blisters.

Sub-acute stage

Greyish or red patches with crusting and scaling.

Chronic stage

Presents with thickened patches, with scaling and increased line markings on the skin (this is called lichenification) from repeated scratching.

There are a host of triggers for eczema, including:

- Climate – extremes of temperature, low humidity.
- Irritants – detergents, wools or other fabrics.
- Infections.
- Environmental allergens – dust mites, pollens, contact allegens for metals or fragrance or pet dander.
- Food allergies – they are a trigger in a minority of eczema patients, especially in babies, commonly to egg, milk and nuts.

Treatment aims are three-fold:

- Treating the active eczema with anti-inflammatory agents – topical steroids or calcineurin inhibitors. The role of these is to help reduce redness and itchiness (i.e. stop the itch–scratch cycle).
- Using moisturisers to maintain the skin barrier.
- Avoiding trigger factors.

Eczema should be treated by your doctor or a dermatologist, but let's discuss the basics of skincare.

Dr V's Formulation Insights

Knowing that itching is the worst symptom of eczema, if you were a formulator, which ingredients would you use and which would you avoid for children when making a product for this skin condition?

I am shocked to know that the vast majority of baby and kids' skincare products contain fragrance.

The other mistake I see are 'natural' products for babies. Essential oils are 'natural' but they are also skin sensitisers. It is better to look at efficiency and the irritant profile of products over being 'natural'. (Please read the section on whether natural products are better than synthetic ones on page 112)

Ingredients to look for:

- Anti-inflammatory: oatmeal, aloe, panthenol
- Humectants: glycerine, urea
- Emollients or occlusives: shea butter, paraffin, petrolatum

Ingredients to avoid:

- Fragrance
- Denatured alcohol
- Essential oils

Eczema skincare routine

Try this routine when eczema is flaring up:

- Ensure showers are lukewarm and short – no more than 5 minutes.
- Avoid bar soaps.
- Use a non-fragranced and hydrating shower gel.
- Use a paraffin shower gel to behave as an occlusive.
- Use non-fragranced body oils, such as sweet almond oil, when the skin is still wet, then pat dry.
- Use a thicker ointment to moisturise instead of creams.

Avoid lotions as the water content is usually too high and the occlusive percentage is lower.

I personally never recommend lotions for skin of colour. We already have fewer ceramides than Caucasian skin, which means our skin is slightly drier. Lotions don't help the situation.

Dealing with a flare up

Topical steroids should be applied in the correct way and the correct quantity as recommended by the doctor. Remember that when used correctly, topical steroids very rarely cause side-effects (such as thinning skin from long-term use, broken capillaries, acne or rosacea). You should start with the lowest potency of steroids, in order to reduce the possibility of other side-effects. Remember, that using occlusives (such as petroleum jelly) will increase the absorption of topical steroids. Different forms of steroids will also affect absorption – for example thick steroid ointment will act as an occlusive, so you get more penetration than with a steroid cream.

You can wrap the area in bandages to act as a second skin. This will hold water in the epidermis, keep infection out and reduce the effects of scratching.

Antihistamines have been shown to relieve itching, and antibiotics can be prescribed for secondary infections (if needed).

Don't forget that eczema means the skin barrier is compromised. Avoid all irritants especially fragrance, essential oils or alcohol.

Dr V's Top Tips on using an emollient:
- Be liberal.
- Use frequently.
- Re-apply at least every 2–3 hours.
- Creams tend to be better tolerated during the day.
- Ointments tend to be better tolerated during the night.

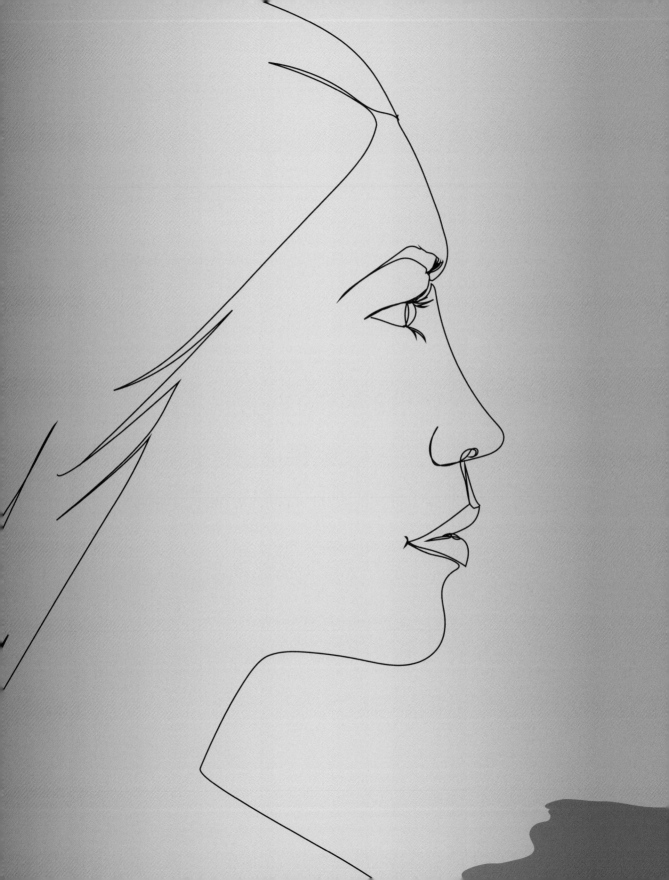

8

Common
SKIN
conditions

Keratosis pilaris (aka chicken skin)

Keratosis pilaris is very common and has a few different names, but it is most often known as 'chicken skin'.

It feels like rough, bumpy skin which is caused by dead skin cells and hard keratin plugging your hair follicles. You might see redness or a burgundy colour from inflammation or if you scratch the area. This happens when too much keratin is produced – generally as an older child or teenager. It also worsens during pregnancy for reasons that are still unclear. Keratin forms a plug in the hair follicle and can also trap hair, leading to the signature bumps of 'chicken skin'.

Keratosis pilaris is found where there are lots of hair follicles, so you'll see it on the upper arms, thighs, buttocks and cheeks. This is why you won't see any 'chicken skin' on the palms or soles, where there are no hair follicles. Keratosis pilaris tends to be worse in winter due to increased TEWL (trans-epidermal water loss), which leads to dehydrated skin. You can take measures to improve its appearance, but you can't cure it, although it may resolve itself by your thirties.

Home remedies

Take a short, warm bath to open pores. Don't luxuriate in long baths as this dehydrates the skin and increases TEWL.

Try some gentle exfoliation with 2% salicylic acid (BHA). The reason being that salicylic acid penetrates the pore to unclog it as it is fat-soluble. You can also add mandelic acid or lactic acid (AHAs), which are water-soluble and work on the epidermis – this will 'brighten' the skin and improve penetration of actives but it won't unclog the pore. It is still debatable if this approach works, however, as often dry skin worsens keratosis pilaris and salicylic acid can lead to further dry skin. I recommend you use one with humectants in it to minimise the chances of this. Also, don't do this until your teenage years; it is too harsh for children.

Hydrate using paraffin-based shower gels to decrease itchiness, then apply thick creams with humectants such as urea and glycerine and emollients such as paraffin.

Use humidifiers to ensure water is drawn from the environment into the skin rather than the other way around. This will decrease itchiness and allow the skin to heal.

A lot of the products on the market are geared to aggressive exfoliation, so you need to take care.

Dry skin + skin of colour + harsh scrubbing = micro tears, worsening irritation and possible hyperpigmentation.

It's better to opt for hydration over exfoliation.

Dr V's Recommendations:

Paula's Choice weightless body treatment 2% BHA (££)

10% urea Eucerin intensive lotion. Hydrates the skin, decreases itchiness and is fragrance free (£)

Oilatum gel, 70% light liquid paraffin (£)

Common mistakes

Avoid scrubbing with a loofah – this can irritate and lead to inflammation. This also only tackles the outer layer of epidermis, not *inside the pore* where the keratin plug has formed.

Also avoid microdermabrasion or deep chemical peels as they irritate and inflame skin, too.

Avoid soap bars as they contain solidifying agents and can clog pores.

Remember, dry skin worsens keratosis pilaris, so please avoid drying alcohols in your skincare.

Avoid known irritants such as fragrance and essential oils.

Keloids

Keloid scarring is when there is overgrowth of tissue outside the boundary of the original wound. There is very little that can be done, scarring may persist and treatment is often limited.

There is no definitive, curative treatment for keloid scarring. Most treatment options will focus on improving the appearance of the scar: to flatten it, make it smaller, or lighter. Generally, dermatologists would offer interlesional triamcilanone injections (ILT) over multiple courses to improve the appearance of the keloid to make it more similar to surrounding skin. Excision (cutting out the keloid) is another method a trained dermatologist might try – however, the risk of this treatment is that a keloid scar is being replaced by another scar, and the keloid could recur. Board-approved plastic surgeons are another port of call for treating keloids and offer a range of treatments.

There has been some evidence of temporary improvement with steroid injections into the scar every few weeks, which may also help control the growth, but avoid peels or trauma to the skin, which can trigger more scarring. Using emollients and silicone gel sheets may help with the uncomfortableness.

Acanthosis nigricans (aka dark, velvety patches on skin)

At the Hyperpigmentation Clinic, a common issue that clients had was Acanthosis nigricans – a skin condition that causes darker patches of skin most often found under the arms and on the back of the neck. Most people affected thought they simply had hyperpigmentation. However, Acanthosis nigricans is more than hyperpigmentation and causes not only darkening of the skin, but thickening of the skin affected, resulting in a 'velvety' texture. It would usually show up in these areas:

Back of the neck   Groin area
Under arm   Back of the knees

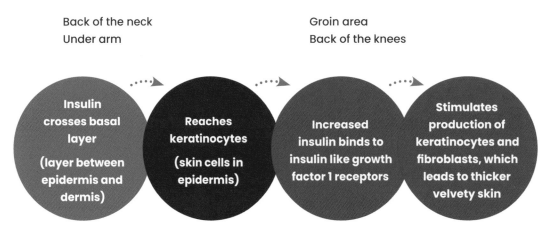

How is Acanthosis nigricans caused?

The most common cause of Acanthosis nigricans is obesity. Over 50% of those who weigh more than double their recommended weight develop Acanthosis nigricans in adulthood.

Acanthosis nigricans also frequently occurs when you have diabetes, as well as being very overweight, which is why it's becoming increasingly common as skin-of-colour communities are being affected more and more by these two issues.

Treatment

You can use gentle peels such as mandelic acid, but until the root cause is fixed, this can only give temporary results.

Avoid lasers in skin of colour as it can burn and lead to more pigmentation.

> **Reducing your weight and exercising more will improve insulin sensitivity, meaning circulating insulin will reduce, which will improve the effects of Acanthosis nigricans.**

Milia around eyes

Milia are seen as small white or yellow bumps under the skin of the eyelids, nose or cheeks. Milia are made of keratin, which gets trapped under the skin. They can grow to 2mm but usually they are tiny, very stubborn and difficult to treat with a normal skincare routine. It is important to note that milia are not clogged pores or a form of acne. They are simple, hard, keratin protein trapped in the skin.

It's not clear what causes milia, although it's potentially due to harsh skin products, dermabrasion or sunburn. As the skin peels in response to the inflammation, bits of epidermis get trapped under skin. This is why I don't think the delicate eye area should ever have a peel. This is a common mistake made when trying to treat dark circles.

How do you treat milia?

These are stuck to the skin, so it is unlikely that any over-the-counter medication will help.

Options to try first include:

Salicylic acid
Vitamin A family

MYTH: You aren't cleansing properly.

MYTH: Steaming your face will remove milia – this may help soften the top layer of skin and make extraction easier by a dermatologist but it won't treat the milia and may lead to irritation of the skin. (I am NOT a fan of steaming the face.)

MYTH: Home remedies – rose water and manuka honey; there is not much clinical evidence to back this up.

How to choose the best professional treatment for skin of colour

De-rooting by a dermatologist, which involves a tiny cut after which the milia are flicked out, can lead to inflammation and pigmentation but the risks are less than other options such as cryotherapy (when the milia are frozen and removed using liquid nitrogen).

Sebaceous filaments

'When I squeeze my skin this white stuff comes out of my pores… It feels so satisfying!' (Ever heard this before?)

This white stuff is actually sebaceous filaments, which are naturally occurring, tube-like structures that fill the walls of your pores. Think of them like straws that direct oil flow to the surface. The purpose of sebaceous filaments is to transport oil to your skin surface and hydrate your skin.

They are a normal part of the skin and you can't get rid of them, but you can minimise their appearance.

There is some confusion between black heads and sebaceous filaments

Sebaceous filaments are normal structures in skin (they line the pores). Over-production of sebum plus dead skin cells can clog the pore and lead to a black head (or white head) developing (see page 170).

Skincare routine

- Use micellar water to remove oil-based dirt.
- Apply oil-soluble salicylic acid at 0.5–2% to regulate sebum production.
- Using a 2–5% niacinamide serum will control sebum production.
- A layer of broad spectrum sunscreen is essential. UV exposure can enlarge pores, making sebaceous filaments more obvious. Look for oil-free or non-comedogenic sunscreens.

Common mistakes:

The American Academy of Dermatology advises against squeezing or extracting. Even if you squeeze the sebaceous filaments or use suction devices to remove them (which are a terrible idea for skin of colour) the filaments will fill up again in just one month.

Squeezing or sucking the skin leads to inflammation, damage of pores, cuts and bruising. Guess what can happen next? Our sensitive melanocytes get very angry and start firing out excess melanin, leading to hyperpigmentation.

It may feel satisfying to extract your sebaceous filaments, but please avoid it, especially with pore vacuums that can cause bruising, pigmentation and permanent damage to your skin.

Please also avoid drying alcohol, comedogenic creams or makeup in your skincare.

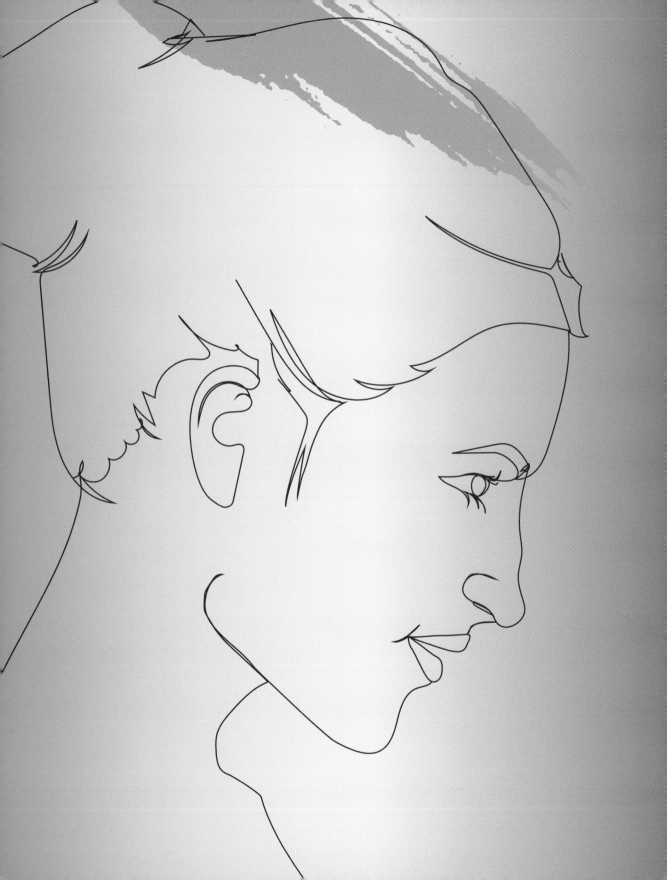

9

HAIR
AND
SKIN

Welcome to the skincare you didn't know you needed. An often-neglected area, this section will show you how to keep your scalp in great condition. And when you have a healthy scalp, you have healthy hair growth!

The scalp

The scalp is full of sebaceous glands, which leads to oily hair and growth of Malassezia, (see page 187). This means we do not want to add oil or conditioner, and in particular essential oils or denatured alcohol, directly to the scalp. For faster, healthier hair growth I recommend using water-based serums with the ingredients **vitamins A, B (biotin), C, D and E**, plus **caffeine, peptides, niacinamide** (sebum control), and anti-inflammatory ingredients such as **allantoin, aloe** and **panthenol**, to be massaged into the scalp. Please also refer to the collagen supplement section on page 96 to learn about how these products can be used to improve hair growth. I prefer you use oils on the hair shaft itself to smooth cuticles, reduce frizz and tangles, which means less breakage during brushing, combing or styling.

When shampooing your hair you want to massage the product into the scalp, which is often inflamed or flaky. Look for fragrance-free formulas with gentle surfactants and lots of humectants (such as **glycerine** or **urea**) and anti-inflammatory ingredients (such as aloe and panthenol).

When conditioning the hair, we want to work from two-thirds of the way down a strand, so that the conditioner makes the hair less tangled and easier to handle. We don't want it on the scalp itself.

When choosing your conditioner, you want to look for emollients. More than this you want to ensure no irritants, especially fragrance, touch the scalp. Fragrance is the number one cause of contact dermatitis. Wash-off products are permitted to use a higher percentage of fragrance, and conditioners use a *lot* of fragrance. This is one reason I prefer to use conditioners only on hair (which is dead), not the sensitive, blood-rich skin of the scalp.

I am a fan of hair masks after showering to seal in proteins such as keratin and emollients to smooth the hair cuticle and minimise hair tangling, silicones to protect from heat styling, UV filters and antioxidants to mop up free radicals that damage the scalp skin. The big mistake I see is people brushing their hair vigorously when it is still wet. When hair is wet, the diameter of the hair strands swells and they are fragile, snapping easily. Always gently comb your hair when it is dry with a wide-tooth comb, which is why I find hair masks excellent as they make this process far less traumatic! Start from the bottom and work your way up. If you have dry or curly hair then I recommend applying a leave in conditioner then using a microfibre towel to cut drying time in half. Your hair will feel damp an hour later but smoother, this is when you can brush your hair from the bottom up to reduce tangles. Don't forget to wash your brushes or combs monthly, too. Sebum and dead skin cells build up on your brush!

The other myth is that you can't shampoo daily – this is not true, especially if you exercise and sweat daily, in which case you must remove the oil from your scalp. However, if you are not exercising getting a sweaty scalp every day then it is better to reduce how often you wash your hair. Water weakens the hair as the strands swell and when hair loss is your biggest issue then you must protect your hair as much as possible. I limit my hair washing to 1-2 times a week.

Please avoid oiling the scalp, I am happy for you to oil the hair, though – the best oils for hair strands include:

- Coconut oil
- Argan oil
- Jojoba oil
- Sweet almond oil

Gentle scalp massage with a water-based serum is thought to stretch the cells of hair follicles, thereby increasing hair thickness. It also improves blood flow, which increases hair growth.

Infra-red light on the scalp can help hair growth if you have viable hair follicles. Usually you wear it for 20 minutes every other day for 4–6 months, then twice a week. You can buy an infra-red helmet online or from specialist providers. (I'm wearing mine right now!)

If you are bald, protect your scalp and please don't forget your sunscreen!

How to treat dandruff and seborrheic dermatitis

What is dandruff?

Dandruff is in its more basic terms patches of oily flakes on the scalp that cause itching. You may see embarrassing white or grey flakes on a black jumper; these flakes are small and confined to the scalp.

What is seborrheic dermatitis?

Seborrheic dermatitis manifests as yellow, greasy scales with mounds on the scalp, with some irritation visible. You can also see red or darker scaly patches on ears, eyebrows, chest and nostrils. It can be extremely itchy.

Dandruff and seborrheic dermatitis might actually be the same condition – but to different degrees. Observational studies have demonstrated seborrheic dermatitis and dandruff leads to duller, thinner, more brittle hair. This is why when you want to grow healthy, luscious hair you NEED to start from healthy scalp skin.

Who gets dandruff or seborrheic dermatitis?

Dandruff is incredibly common. A broad survey of 1,400 multi-ethnic adults showed that roughly 60–90% of adults have dandruff.

Dandruff can recur and can also become chronic, which is thought to be because of this cycle:

- Increased oil is released from your scalp's sebaceous glands
- Increase of yeast, aka Malassezia
- This means your skin reacts to Malassezia even faster next time.

What is happening

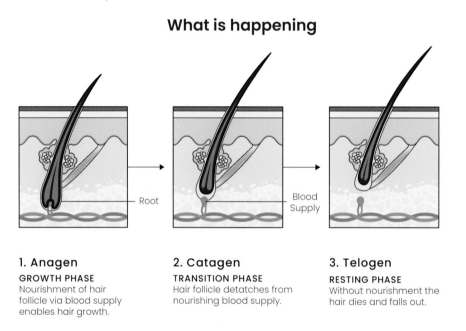

1. Anagen
GROWTH PHASE
Nourishment of hair follicle via blood supply enables hair growth.

2. Catagen
TRANSITION PHASE
Hair follicle detatches from nourishing blood supply.

3. Telogen
RESTING PHASE
Without nourishment the hair dies and falls out.

What are the treatment options?

Dandruff and seborrheic dermatitis irritate and inflame the skin of the scalp. Dandruff treatment is big business, and some products are more effective at treating the condition than others, but some will only tackle the problem on a short-term basis. The majority of shampoos (including anti-dandruff shampoos) contain fragrance, essential oils or masking agents. These are good for your nose but BAD for sensitive-scalp skin. I have no idea why they do this but please read the ingredients carefully (see opposite). If OTC products don't work, then see your GP or a dermatologist for prescription-strength products.

Anti-fungal agents:

- 2% Ketoconazole shampoo is an anti-fungal against Malassezia with an anti-inflammatory effect.

- This is one of my favourite options if there is irritation or sensitivity. Recommended use is twice a week for a minimum of 4 weeks. I use this shampoo indefinitely to keep my seborrheic dermatitis at bay.
- Zinc pyrithione kills yeast overgrowth
- Topical Calcineurin inhibitors such as primecrolimus 1% and tacrolimus 0.03% should be used more for facial seborrheic dermatitis

Exfoliating agents

Salicylic acid and coal tar softens and improves the scaling, which improves the penetration of anti-fungals.

Anti-inflammatory agents

Steroid creams can be used in the short term for a severe flare up. They should not be used long term, though.

Important to note:

This is a condition that will return once you stop your anti-fungal treatment.

Treatment

Start with an easy to use anti-fungal shampoo such as 2% Ketoconazole. Leave this on the scalp for 5–10 minutes before rinsing off thoroughly.

Recommended ingredients and ideal percentages

Zinc pyrithione

0.3–2% in shampoo
0.1–0.25% leave-in products

Selenium sulfide

0.6–1%

Salicylic acid

1.8–2%

Coal tar

0.5–5% reduces number and size of epidermal cells and reduced proliferation

Sulfur

2–5%

Dr V's Dandruff Shampoo Recommendations:

Nizoral (£)
Alpecin (£)
DHS Sal shampoo (£)
Sebclair (£)

DHS Tar Shampoo (£)
T/Sal Neutrogena therapeutic shampoo (fragrance-free version) (£)

Facial hair

Facial hair removal can be the bane of many women's lives, from the teens onwards! Figuring out how to remove hair and keep skin in good condition can be a tricky balancing act.

My mum and grandma were both blessed with hairless faces and bodies. My father, on the other hand, is particularly hairy. Guess who I took after? I can definitely say that hair removal is a topic I can speak about with authority and experience.

Typically, there are four locations on the face where hairs grow and which cause the most concern for women when it comes to hair removal.

Upper lips

Eyebrows

Chin

Cheeks

The most important thing for skin of colour is to have minimal inflammation or irritation of the skin.

Any burning can result in PIH.

Ideally you want to remove hair from the root to reduce the chance of ingrown hair. When I tweezer my eyebrows (in between threading, I know, very bad, my beautician tells me off every time) it leads to hairs breaking, which either gives my brows a green hue or a black dot, neither of which can be covered well with makeup!

My favourite options:

Threading – this is best for eyebrows, upper lip and chin. You may find the cheeks too large an area to thread, I know I do (I'm also a pathetic baby who tears up with every pass of the twisted thread). I remember my first eyebrow threading experience. I barely got one brow done, then refused to do the other one!

Tweezing – is also a good option for eyebrows – take care not to break the hair, you need to pull the whole hair shaft out.

Epilators – do the same thing as threading but treat bigger areas, for example cheeks. This can be painful, though. You have been warned!

These three forms don't use chemicals, so there is minimal chance of an allergic reaction or chemical burns.

Waxing – Hot wax is better for coarse hair on cheeks than strip wax.

Please note: This can cause irritation, and can also lead to breakage of the hair shaft, which can lead to an ingrown hair.

Avoid waxing if you:

- have sensitive skin
- are using a vitamin A product
- have done a chemical peel in the last 4 weeks
- are on antibiotics that sensitise the skin
- are prone to breakouts

I would avoid home hot-waxing kits, especially for skin of colour, as the temperature gauge is not always accurate which can result in PIH.

Side-effects of waxing:

- It is normal to have some redness or flushed skin and irritation.
- If little pimples are forming this could be inflammation of a hair follicle, called folliculitis.
- If you're experiencing swelling and pain, it could be an allergy to the wax causing contact dermatitis. If it happens once, at a later date, do a patch test in a discrete area such as on your forearm or behind the ear.
- Whenever you are removing hair, if the area is inflamed, use ice in a clean cloth on the skin afterwards to soothe and vasoconstrict to prevent inflammatory mediators flooding the area.

Shaving the face; Dermaplaning – when a blade is used to remove hair and exfoliate the top layer of skin – is painless but it's a myth that hair grows back thicker after this. Once a hair has been cut, it is no longer tapered (thick at the root, fine at the tip). Because it is cut somewhere in the middle, the tip is rough rather than fine, so the hair grows back sharper not thicker.

Shaving tips:

- Shave skin that has first been soaked skin in water.
- Use a pre-shave oil to decrease PIH from razor burns.
- Pass the razor over the area only one time to minimise irritation.

Hair-removal creams – Depilatory creams (hair-removal creams) contain alkaline substances that break down keratin (protein bonds) in the hair below the skin's surface. Examples of these substances include:

- calcium thioglycolate
- potassium thioglycolate
- sodium thioglycolate
- strontium sulfide

The BEST part of this form of hair removal is that it is painless, but it's also better than shaving as it breaks the hair under the skin's surface so it takes longer to grow back. Shaving does leave a sharp end, which makes it feel prickly when it grows back, but hair-removal creams lead to tapered, softer hair ends.

Using a cream is my preferred method for first hair removal of the upper lip, under arm or lower leg. Beware, though, it can be smelly and messy and can lead to patchy hair removal if it is done on a large area as well.

Please take care not to leave on your skin longer than the recommended time, to reduce the chance of irritation. Not following recommended timings can lead to skin burns and inflammation.

Laser hair removal – skin of colour requires a longer wavelength laser, so energy is focused on the hair follicle in the dermis rather than the higher basal layer where melanocytes live. This is why we recommend ND:YAG lasers for darker skin tones. There are risks with all laser use of burns and hyperpigmentation but this is the best option for us. Please see page 124 for further information.

Skin procedures

Let's discuss common skin procedures you may opt for in a clinic.

Microneedling

I personally love microneedling for skin of colour as it causes minimal inflammation, so the risk of post inflammatory hyperpigmentation is reduced.

Dimensions of a derma roller

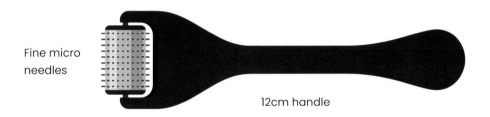

Fine micro needles

12cm handle

Micro needles are usually 0.2–0.3mm in length, depending on which area of the body you are working on and the purpose they are being used for.

For example:

Home use – for a facial derma roller for fine lines use 0.2mm needles.
For stretch marks on the body you may prefer a 3mm derma roller.

How it works

Microneedling causes controlled micro-injury with minimal damage to the epidermis.

> *Examination of skin after four microneedling sessions one month apart showed a 400% increase in collagen and elastin six months after completion.*

It also improves scar tissue as it breaks down old scar strands allowing blood to be restored to old hardened scars, this encourages collagen formation in a regular lattice pattern. In the clinic we use microneedling to treat dark circles.

First, we prime the area with a vitamin A, C and E cream to minimise any chances of pigmentation. Then we clean and topically numb the skin using lidocaine and prilocaine.

As we derma roll the periorbital area (eyelid and under eye) we use a narrow-head derma roller. The derma roller is rolled in each area in multiple directions over about 15 passes in total per cm squared.

If you go to a clinic just for dermarolling, then your practitioner may just finish the treatment at this point with saline or cool the area. As we are doing the treatment for the purposes of treating dark circles, we use this temporary channel opening to apply soothing tyrosinase inhibitors to reduce dark circles.

We advise the patient to wear large sunglasses going home, to use sunscreen around the eyes and avoid use of makeup for a couple of days.

Collagen can be laid down for 3–6 months after treatments, so you may see results even six months after your last treatment.

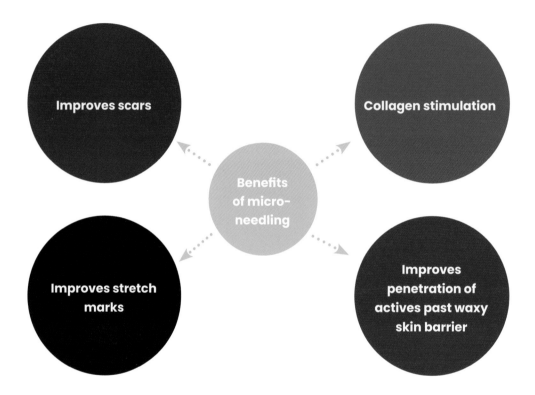

Avoid derma-rolling if you have:

- Cystic acne (see page 184)
- A tendency to keloid – which means you have had hypertrophic scars (an overgrowth of scar tissue leading to a raised scar) in the past
- A damaged and/or irritated skin barrier
- Any infection of the skin
- Any clotting issues

How to choose micro-needle length

I would reserve the 1.5mm-plus needles for professionals rather than for home use as these are painful and you need sufficient numbing first.

- 0.2mm – best for getting ingredients deeper into the skin past the waxy barrier. I use this length for a deep wrinkle concentrate I made for my crows' feet and laughter lines (marionette lines) (home use).
- 0.5mm – this enters the dermis to stimulate collagen (anti-ageing).
- 1.5mm – penetrates the dermis deeper to break up scar tissue and encourage 'normal' formation of collagen.
- 1.5–3mm – these are for thicker body skin, mainly for stretch marks.

How to take care of your home derma roller

Each derma roller typically can be used by a single person 2–3 times a week, up to 100 times.

After you use the roller, wash it in hot water and let it air dry in its case so the head is not touching anything. Do not use a towel as fibres get stuck on the needles.

Some like to soak their micro-needle head in isopropyl alcohol for about 10 minutes, then rinse it in hot water and let it air dry.

Treating the skin after dermarolling

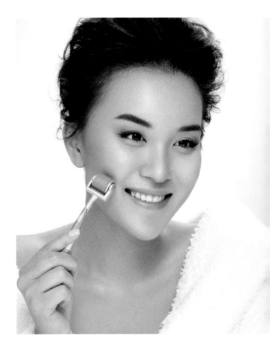

Once you have finished dermarolling, treat your skin. Avoid any acids, which will aggravate your skin. I make myself a retinaldehyde deep-wrinkle concentrate to apply over the dermarolled area. As vitamin A is dehydrating, I also incorporate ceramides and humectants, and as it can still be irritating, I love to use aloe and Panthenol at the same time.

As I am trying to stimulate collagen, I also use tetrahexyldecyl ascorbate and peptides.

These are the sorts of ingredients I would love you to use after dermarolling for anti-ageing or for post-acne scar texture treatment.

Facial steaming

Before my wedding, when I was doing everything I could think of to have the perfect skin for my special day, I listened to my beautician and got my face steamed. I had no idea what the pros or cons were, I just followed suit and she proceeded to scrape my nose – which was very painful! Looking back, and knowing what I know now, I am disappointed that I was 'swayed by the marketing', which could have damaged my skin.

How much of this is actually true?

MYTH: Steam opens pores and releases dirt.

TRUTH: It may open pores and soften the skin but steam cannot enter the pore to unclog anything.

MYTH: Steam releases any C. acnes bacteria trapped in the sebum.

TRUTH: Comedones – white heads, black heads and pimples – are formed by a sticky mixture of sebum and dead skin cells. Steam is unable to remove this. You need a fat-soluble acid such as salicylic acid to do this 'job'. Under the sticky plug, is the anaerobic C. acnes bacteria, so how can steam 'release' the bacteria if it cannot penetrate the plug?

MYTH: Steam is hydrating.

TRUTH: It opens pores but it increases trans-epidermal water loss, which actually dehydrates the skin. There is more water evaporation from the skin.

MYTH: Steam improves permeability of actives.

TRUTH: If you want to improve permeability, use a hydrating toner and exfoliate as the safest way to increase permeability, as you are removing the top layer of compacted dead skin cells. Please read the chapter on how to exfoliate skin of colour.

MYTH: It is relaxing to use, especially with essential oils or fragrance.

TRUTH: It is a mistake to combine steam with essential oils or fragrance. They both lead to skin sensitivity and potential contact dermatitis, which will lead to dry and inflamed skin.

MYTH: Use steam and acids together to penetrate skin deeper.

TRUTH: Let's go back to our chemistry days at school...Water molecules are constantly colliding and splitting into positively charged $H+$ ion and $OH-$ ions.

Remember:

$$H^+ + OH^- = H_2O$$

(Called 'Auto-dissociation' of water)

We can only measure the pH of a solution that has H+ ions. This means water MUST be the solvent.

Measuring the Hydrogen Ion Activity will tell us if the solution is acidic, alkaline or neutral.

This is why we rub in a gentle acid such as mandelic acid in a clinic setting to generate heat and lower the pH. If you add heat to glycolic acid, however, it can lead to burns and PIH in skin of colour.

This is why I would never combine an acid that is already known to cause PIH in skin of colour with heat. It will lead to much headache. Some people will be fine, but remember my aim is always to get zero per cent burns in skin of colour.

My final thoughts on steaming:

As you probably know by now, I am not a fan of actively inflaming skin, especially skin of colour.

I understand the vasodilation (the expanding of blood vessels) gives you a 'flush' appearance that you can mistake as a 'healthy glow' but as this is a temporary dilating of blood vessels, the repercussions aren't worth it. Redness and swelling can exacerbate rosacea, eczema and melasma.

There is also the possibility of 'overdoing it' and burning the skin.

So, what are we supposed to do instead, Dr V?

I prefer you do the opposite and cool the skin, to decrease inflammation and puffiness. Both of these factors increase with age.

I would also recommend you use the correct ingredients to unclog pores – salicylic acid or clay masks.

For a long-term benefit, it's better to exfoliate and hydrate your skin correctly. If you like the idea of fragrance around you as you treat your skin, I suggest you use fragrance candles and spray perfume in the room, but please avoid using this on the skin directly.

NEVER use acids with heat on the skin.

KEEPING YOUR SKIN CALM AND HAPPY IS ESSENTIAL FOR SKIN OF COLOUR.

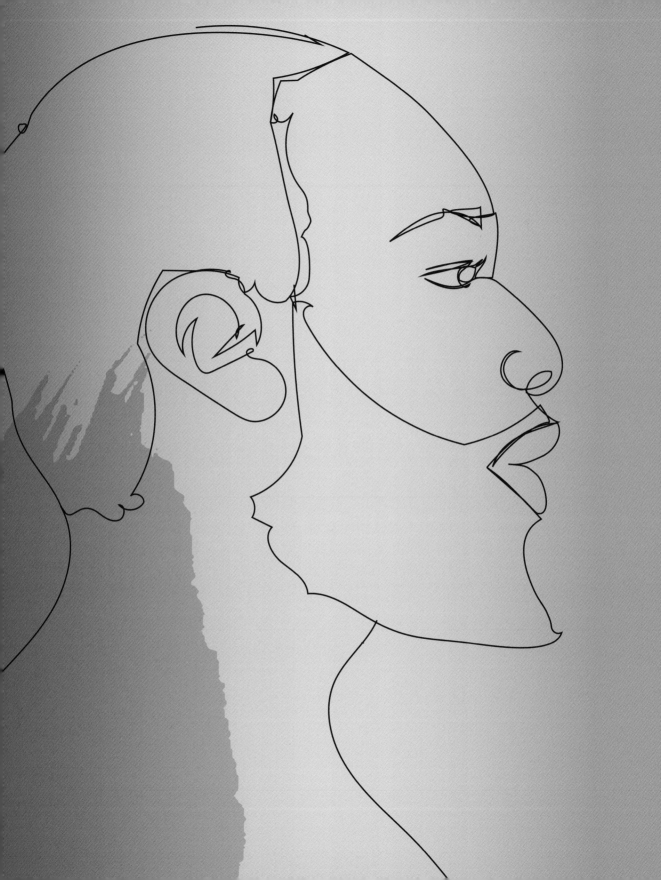

10

SKINCARE
for men

We know that skin of colour needs particular love and care, and that's what *Skin Revolution* is all about. But what are the differences in skincare between men and women? This chapter is all about the men in our skin-of-colour family – because your skin deserves specific care for your needs, too!

There are many conflicting studies about male versus female skin, from skin elasticity and pH to micro-circulation and hydration, but the majority of studies support the following points that can help you understand your skin better.

- Men generally have higher testosterone levels and so produce 2–4 times more sebum than women. This leads to oilier skin, larger pores and also more prolonged acne along with possible scarring on the face, chest, back and shoulders. (See more about how to treat back acne on page 185.)

- Men have a 20% thicker dermis compared to women, which means they don't wrinkle in the same way. Men tend to get deep expression lines, not the superficial wrinkles that women are affected with. Men also tend to have a larger muscle mass, which means that their facial wrinkles get even deeper. (See more about anti-ageing on page 148.)

- The dermis on men's skin (second layer of skin which is supplied with blood flow) is more sensitive to environmental assault compared to women, especially UV rays. Unfortunately, men are generally not as vigilant with applying SPF50 as women are. I hope this book helps change your approach to using sunscreen – see more about how to choose a sunscreen on page 66.

- If you shave your facial hair daily, you might find that initially the skin looks brighter, as you are essentially exfoliating the top layer of dead skin. However, you are actually inflicting daily repeated trauma and inflammation in the process. Testosterone actually slows repair of wounds and the following ingredients in the most popular aftershaves make irritation worse:

Alcohol
Fragrance
Essential oils
Menthol

Some myth-busting on wearing aftershaves:

MYTH: 'I feel like I smell good, which makes me feel good.'

TRUTH: Wear a nice-smelling mist or perfume on your clothes, go to town! But leave your poor skin alone, it can't yell at you to stop.

MYTH: 'I feel like it is closing the wounds.'

TRUTH: You aren't, if anything you are delaying the wound from healing and fragrance is the number one cause of contact dermatitis. In aftershaves, fragrance is high up on the INCI (ingredients) list.

MYTH: 'I feel like the sting is killing bacteria.'

TRUTH: That sting is from a denatured alcohol and menthol. Denatured alcohol is drying as it evaporates quickly and menthol is a skin sensitiser. I wouldn't apply these ingredients to inflamed skin.

MYTH: 'It hasn't done any visible damage so why stop?'

TRUTH: Your skin is good at hiding minor irritation, but over a long period of time it leads to skin dehydration and premature ageing.

What is the best cleanser for men?

Men tend to have oiler skin than women, which is why I would recommend a gentle, non-fragranced salicylic acid face wash or one with niacinamide in it.

What is the best moisturiser for men?

Although the male dermis is thicker, it is more prone to damage, which is why I would recommend non-irritating antioxidants; so for both morning and evening, use **green tea extract, resveratrol** and **vitamin E.**

Men's skin tends to be more sensitive, especially if you are shaving regularly, which is why I recommend anti-inflammatory ingredients such as aloe and panthenol.

A star ingredient you may want to look for is potassium azeloyl diglycinate, which is anti-ageing, brightening and controls sebum. Niacinamide will also help with this but I like the percentage at 2–5% for daily use.

Men still need the same ceramides, peptides, humectants and occlusives in their skincare routine, too.

What is the best sunscreen for men?

If you are shaving regularly, then I recommend mineral SPF50 sunscreen with zinc oxide for its anti-inflammatory benefits. Please see how to choose the best sunscreen on page 66.

Step-by-step skincare routine for men who shave

From my experience, men aren't as eager to follow a 7-step nightly routine as women are – and this includes my husband, who just wants the basics to 'get the job done in the least amount of time'.

I recommend those who shave follow this routine:

Note: Please see page 30 to find out how to identify your skin type.

 AM ROUTINE

> **Step 1:** Wash with micellar gel wash (with or without niacinamide) if you have normal or dry skin, or with salicylic acid wash if you have oily skin.
> **Step 2:** Moisturise with a non-fragranced moisturiser with antioxidants, anti-inflammatories and potassium azeloyl diglycinateor niacinamide ideally, and with ceramides and peptides.
> **Step 3:** Finally, apply sunscreen: mineral SPF50.

🌙 **PM ROUTINE**

> **Step 1:** Wash with benzoyl peroxide if you have acne-prone skin, your skin will be less likely to be irritated if this is done at night; or follow your morning washing routine for other skin types.
> **Step 2:** Moisturise with a non-fragranced moisturiser with antioxidants, anti-inflammatories and potassium azeloyl diglycinate or niacinamide ideally, and with ceramides and peptides.

Do you feel like you have sensitive skin?

Yes (369 responses) **No** (104 responses)

78%	22%

Have you had a reaction or feel sensitive to fragranced alcohol aftershave?

Yes (255 responses) **No** (80 responses)

76%	24%

Do you wish skincare was simpler?

Yes (352 responses) **No** (53 responses)

88%	12%

Polls performed on men of colour

Dr V's Formulation Insights

This poll tells me we need to keep it simple by using:

1. A fragrance-free aftershave and a hydrating, soothing, anti-inflammatory, anti-pigmentation gel moisturiser.

2. A hydrating, fragrance-free, denatured alcohol-free mineral sunscreen (zinc oxide) SPF50 with pH-neutral antioxidants and niacinamide.

So if I were to put my formulation hat on to solve the problem of best aftershave product, I would create a cooling gel with the following ingredient categories:

- Anti-inflammatory
- Humectants
- Antioxidants to reduce premature ageing and improve skin repair
- Anti-hyperpigmentation (for ingrown hairs/PIH razor burns)

Common mistakes in men's skincare routines

Ask around and you'll find most men are making the same mistakes when it comes to their skincare routine, and it doesn't help you when people are giving the wrong advice online, too. So, here are a few things that I see friends, family and patients doing on a regular basis:

Using hand soap to wash the face – you need a hydrating micellar gel wash.

Using harsh scrubs aggressively – this leads to micro tears and damage to the skin barrier.

Using an alcohol aftershave to 'kill bacteria' – there aren't any dangerous bacteria on the skin to kill and alcohol actually slows the wound-healing process. Imagine having inflamed skin and then adding a drying ingredient and fragrance (the number one cause of contact dermatitis)? This is a combination for sensitivity. I have witnessed men literally slapping their faces with aftershave to ensure a burning sensation was taking place. This is a huge 'no'!

Not using moisturiser – moisturiser creates a healing environment for the skin to repair.

Not using SPF50 – zinc oxide in sunscreens is soothing and prevents antioxidants from ageing the skin.

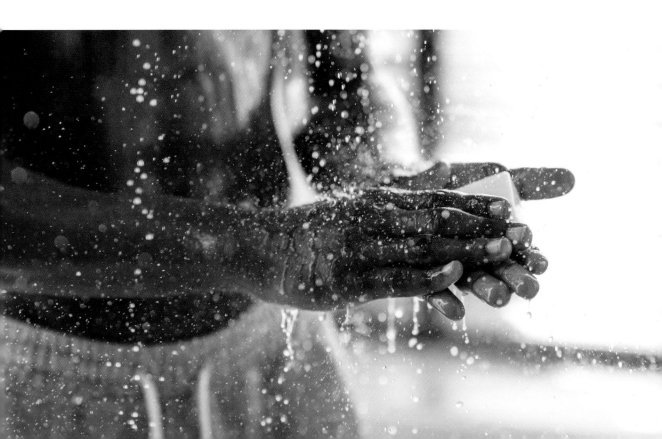

Skincare for men with beards

Facial hair demands a slightly different skincare routine because the skin is hidden, but just because you can't see it, doesn't mean there aren't problems. Some of the issues that men with facial hair experience on the skin beneath a beard include acne, ingrown hair, dandruff and itchiness.

Mythbusting common assumptions about skincare and beards:

MYTH: Using a bar soap on the face is fine.

TRUTH: Bar soap is too alkali for skin on the face. It will strip and dry the skin.

- Please use a gentle cleanser that fits your skin type.
- If you have normal and dry skin, a non-franced micellar gel wash is fine; for oily skin use a salicylic acid face wash.
- If you have acne under your beard use a benzoyl peroxide face wash.

MYTH: You can't exfoliate skin under a beard.

TRUTH: You can and should exfoliate, especially if you have curly thick hair which curls back into the skin causing an ingrown hair.

- I prefer chemical exfoliation over physical or enzyme, especially if skin is irritated from an ingrown hair. I love lactic and mandelic acid for skin of colour. Use it on whole face, including on the skin under your beard.
- If you have oily and acne skin opt for a 2% salicylic acid, leave-on exfoliant.

MYTH: You can't moisturise skin under a beard.

TRUTH: Moisturisation is essential to prevent flaky, dry skin under your beard. There are different options depending on your skin type:

- If you have oily and acne-prone skin use a non-fragranced gel moisturiser or a beard conditioner; for normal and dry skin use a non-fragranced beard oil.
- Massage your moisturiser into the skin beneath the facial hair as the beard may block hydration.

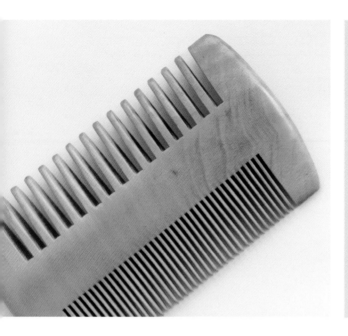

Dr V's Top Tips on Beard Care:

I recommend using a wide-tooth comb to detangle your bead and exfoliate the skin beneath.

If you get beard dandruff (seborrheic dermatitis) use ketoconazole shampoo twice a week; it is a relapsing condition so I wouldn't stop.

Avoid stroking your beard, as you are transferring bacteria to the face.

Daily step-by-step routine

AM ROUTINE

Step 1: Wash (according to your skin type):
  Oily or acne-prone skin – a salicylic acid face wash.
  Normal or dry skin – a micellar gel wash.
Step 2: Moisturise (massage into the beard to reach skin) with a non-fragranced fatty moisturiser.
Step 3: Finish with an SPF50 sunscreen.

PM ROUTINE

Step 1: Wash (according to your skin type):
  Oily or acne-prone skin – a salicylic acid face wash.
  Normal or dry skin – a micellar gel wash.
Step 2: Moisturise (massage into the beard to reach skin) with a NAFE SAFE beard oil if you have dry or normal skin (No Alcohol, Fragrance, Essential oil) or a fatty moisturiser such as Cetraben or Cerave.
Step 3: Use a wide-tooth comb to brush your beard 1–2 times a week to exfoliate.

How to shave

It sounds obvious, but there is a right way to shave, and so many men rush the process, causing damage to their skin. The aim is to cut hair from the beard and stubble as close as possible without causing skin irritation, inflammation or ingrown hairs.

The problem is that beard hair differs from person to person and hair to hair. This includes:

diameter of hair shaft
density and stiffness

direction of growth
low hair growth angle to skin

Additional problems include:

fast beard-hair growth

So, let's look at these issues one by one and how you can solve them.

Diameter of hair shaft – this problem results in men applying more force in shorter strokes and 're-doing' areas of the face. This all results in more irritation and inflammation.

Beard hair has more cuticle layers than hair on the head, which means the diameter of beard hair is double that of scalp hair. This requires more pressure during shaving. This affects electric shaving less than blade shaving.

Density and stiffness – a dry beard is very stiff and will cause too much irritation to cut. This is why it is important to hydrate the hairs for a few minutes before shaving. Stiffness almost halves after 4 minutes and reduces the cutting force.

Fast beard hair growth – there are three main phases of hair growth:

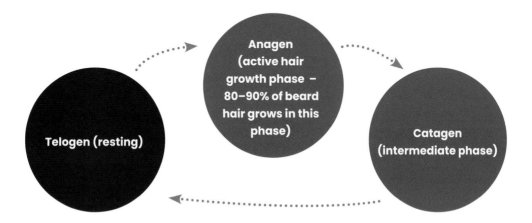

Beard hair grows at about 0.3–0.5mm per day. This dictates how often you shave, depending on how fast your own hair growth is.

Low hair angle – any angle less than 45 degrees is hard to cut. This tends to be worse on the neck, which leads to more inflammation, ingrown hairs and hyperpigmentation for skin of colour men.

The skin is not even – there are contours from chin to the neck, which makes shaving difficult. This is one reason men find shaving the neck trickier.

78% of males reported have skin sensitivity – this was the result of a poll conducted on 473 candidates. Skin surrounding the follicle is very sensitive to inflammation, and when inflammation occurs, we have cells called 'mast cells' that release chemicals leading to pain, swelling and inflammation. This process can be triggered from shaving, which is one of the reasons for irritation and sensitivity after shaving.

How to shave to minimise irritation – follow these simple steps to have a more pleasant and less painful shaving experience!

Step 1: To soften hair, you need to hydrate skin and facial hair for a few minutes. I recommend 4 minutes to hit peak hair softness, which is why shaving after a shower is best.

Step 2: Use a fragrance-free, hydrating shaving cream or gel. Avoid using any irritants before, during or after shaving – don't exfoliate or use acids just before or after. Don't use fragrance or alcohol-based products. Don't use essential oils.

Step 3: Shave in the direction of hair growth, not against the grain, as hair is stiff and you want to cause minimal trauma. Wash the razor after each stroke as there is a build-up of skin and hair on the blade, which stops a sharp cut on the next pass. Use a new blade after seven uses – always keep a sharp blade.

Pseudofolliculitis barbae, or ingrown hair of the beard – this is a chronic inflammatory condition affecting mainly black men and is characterised by curly facial hair growing parallel out of the follicle, then circling back and re-piercing the skin. This is called extra follicular penetration – simply known as ingrown hair.

The body reacts as if a foreign body has entered the skin, with a full inflammatory response complete with swelling, pain and, in males of skin of colour, hyperpigmentation usually results. This is because any form of inflammation leads to hyperpigmentation in skin of colour, the melanocytes (melanin-producing cells) are large and easily triggered.

Have you had ingrown hairs?

Yes (300 responses)   **No** (85 responses)

| 78% | 22% |

Have you had razor burns leading to pigmentation?

Yes (264 responses)   **No** (93 responses)

| 74% | 26% |

Dr V's Interpretation: Men feel a lot of sensitivity after shaving – 78% is a high percentage. Of course, the degree of sensitivity will vary, but it is still an important issue to be aware of. In addition, 76% getting irritation after using a fragranced alcohol aftershave makes me say 'stop using it altogether'. It does you no favours and makes the skin more irritable and dry.

78% of skin-of-colour men getting ingrown hairs is also incredibly high and makes me want to suggest nd:YAG laser just on the neck to break the cycle and allow hyperpigmentation to recover.

74% of skin-of-colour men getting razor burns leading to hyper-pigmentation makes me think that men need a cooling, antioxidant, anti-inflammatory moisturiser with tyrosinase inhibitors.

What should you do?

- Avoid all allergens and irritants. This includes fragrance, denatured alcohol and essential oils.
- Ensure there are no other causes for these symptoms, such as contact dermatitis acne or seborrheic dermatitis.
- We have changed how we manage Pseudofolliculitis barbae once it arises and now we recommend softening hair with warm water and using a hydrating fragrance-free cleanser (micellar gel).
- Multi-razor blades are recommended over a single-blade razor. Ensure the blade is sharp and replaced often.

- Shave daily with light strokes in the direction of hair growth with one pass, not multiple passes.
- Hydration after shaving with non-fragranced moisturiser is now advised.
- In severe cases, anti-inflammatory creams such as steroids may be prescribed.
- You could also try a different form of hair removal, such as an epilator or laser, if shaving is causing severe Pseudofolliculitis barbae.

As a man with ingrown hairs would you consider nd:YAG laser hair removal?

YES (91 responses)   **NO** (80 responses)

| 53% | 47% |

When I asked those who said No to laser why they answered that, the two top responses were:

- It's an expensive procedure.
- They still wanted the option of growing a beard. (Important to note: *There may be a way to just remove hair on the ingrown neck and still be able to grow a beard. It would depend on the location of the hair.*)

If you want to shave after having a beard for a while, I have a few tips for you:

- The skin below will be lighter.
- The skin may be more sensitive as it hasn't been shaved for a while.
- After a shower, hair is softer, so take advantage of this and trim the beard to get as close as possible. Use a shaving cream to minimise irritation and a single sharp blade to minimise razor burns or ingrown hairs. Wash the face with lukewarm water and moisturise well. The skin needs to be hydrated as shaving is essentially mechanical exfoliation for the first time in a while and you want to create a healing environment for the skin.

Sunscreen:
I would want an anti inflammatory mineral (zinc oxide) sunscreen invisible on skin of colour with UV stable tyrosinase inhibitors to tackle pigmentation from ingrown hairs.

TAKING CARE OF MY SKIN IS TAKING CARE OF MYSELF.

Dr V's recommended products for men:

Cleanser:

Simple micellar gel wash (£)

Moisturiser:

Cerave (£), Cetraben (£)

Beard oil:

Simply Great Beard Oil – Unscented (£)
Ranger Unscented Beard Oil (£)
Prophet and Tools Unscented Beard Oil (£)
Badass Beard Oil – Secret Agent (£££)
Bossman Unscented Beard Oil (££)
Zeus Unscented Beard Oil (££)
The Gentlemen's Beard Unscented Beard Oil (£££)

Shaving creams:

Executive Shaving Fragrance Free Shaving Cream (££)
Every Man Jack Shave Cream Sensitive Skin Fragrance free (£)
Vanicream shaving cream (££)
Bull dog sensitive shave cream (£)

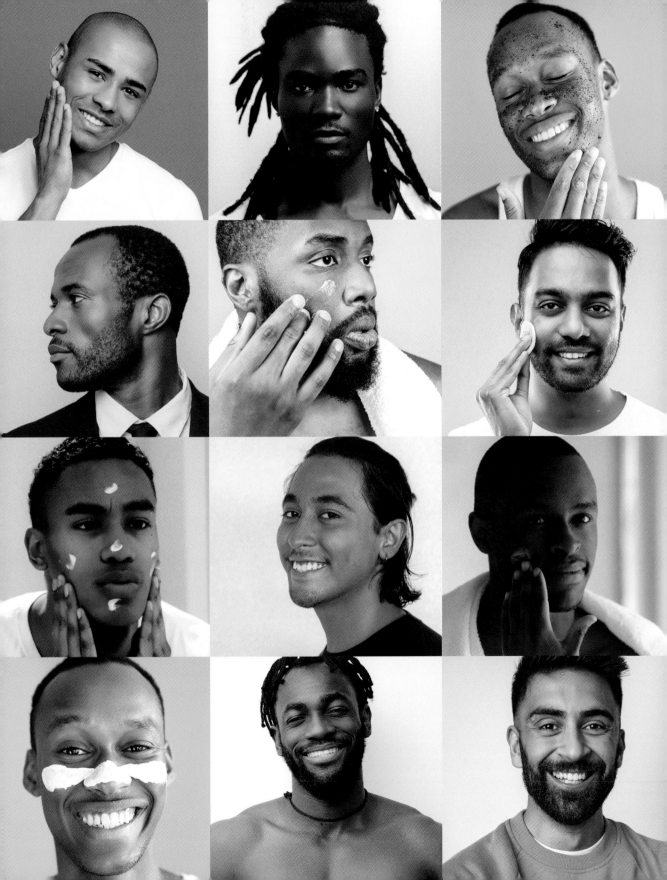

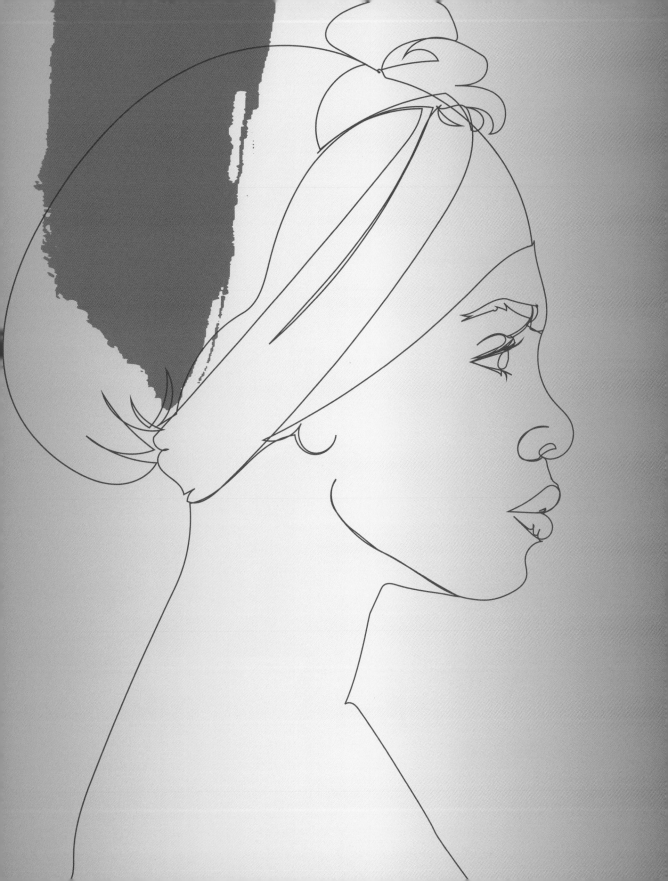

11

Pregnancy
SKINCARE

An Instagram poll suggested that 45–75% of pregnant women with skin of colour develop melasma, which appears as dark brown patches on the cheeks, forehead and upper lip.

Melasma during pregnancy is very common and is also known as chloasma.

I had melasma before pregnancy and I knew it was likely to get worse during pregnancy, so I was obsessive with my sunscreen application every 2 hours. This habit stuck and I carry a bottle of SPF50 in my handbag at all times – in addition to my anti-melasma sunglasses and a scrunched-up UPF50 wide-brimmed hat.

The most common area for melasma is the face, and melasma can show up in the below formations:

- Centro-facial – in over 60% of those affected it shows up on the forehead, upper lip, nose, chin and cheeks.
- Malar – 20% experience it on the cheeks and nose only.
- Mandibular – 16% have it on their jaw .

Women of colour are more prone to melasma during pregnancy, as our melanocytes are larger and easily triggered. The exact pathology is unclear, but it tends to start during the second and third trimesters and is worse in summer or near the equator, where the UV index is higher.

On a positive note, 90% of melasma will resolve within one year of giving birth. If after a year it has not improved, you may need to use higher-strength tyrosinase inhibitors (please read the melasma section on page 119).

Prevention of melasma

Having melasma can lead to much distress, especially as it can take up to a year to clear after pregnancy. This is why prevention is vital by using a broad-spectrum SPF50.

UV exposure is everything, especially when you are already susceptible to pigmentation.

Look at the UV index before leaving the house and always make sure you are carrying the following in your handbag:

- Mineral sunscreen is recommended over chemical sunscreen[6].
- Wear large anti-melasma sunglasses.
- Wide-brimmed hat to minimise direct UV.

> Don't forget SPF50 relates to UVB (rays that burn).
>
> You need broad spectrum for UVA protection (rays that age).

(−) **Anti-melasma ingredients to avoid during pregnancy:**

Vitamin A – we do not have enough data on large cohorts to encourage topical retinoid use. There are published case reports of birth defects associated with topical tretinoin use.

Hydroquinone – as it can be systemically absorbed through the skin.

Over 2% salicylic acid or any other mid or deep chemical peels – due to dermal penetration.

Chemical sunscreens – most chemical sunscreens enter the blood stream and breast milk. There are no long-term studies to assess the safety of this. This is one of the main reasons I recommend mineral sunscreen for our children and for ourselves.

(+) **Anti-melasma ingredients to use during pregnancy:**

Antioxidants: vitamin C, E, green tea extract, resveratrol.

Tyrosinase inhibitors: azelaic acid.

Melanosome transfer interrupter: niacinamide.

AHAs: e.g. mandelic acid and lactic acid.

Mineral zinc oxide sunscreen.

Anti-ageing, pregnancy skincare routine

The average age of pregnancy is increasing from generation to generation. My grandmother had her first baby in her early twenties, my mum had me in her mid-twenties and I had my children in my late twenties and early thirties. This means that for me the ageing process was well under way compared to my grandmother, who looked so young holding my mum as a baby.

This means our skincare needs during pregnancy have also changed.

$(-)$ **Anti-ageing ingredients we avoid during pregnancy include:**

Retinoids (vitamin A family)

Glycolic acid (jury is still out on this AHA during pregnancy)

Chemical sunscreens

High-strength salicylic acid

Liquorice root

Hydroquinone

Alpha arbutin

This rules out a lot of anti-ageing creams!

$(+)$ **Anti-ageing actives can you use:**

Vitamin C

Vitamin E

Co enzyme Q10

Hyaluronic acid

Ceramides

Peptides

Mineral sunscreens, such as zinc oxide

Dr V's Formulation Insights

My skincare aims during pregnancy were to prevent belly stretch marks, keep my melasma at bay and improve my fine lines.

I searched for a product with the ingredients I needed:

- Vitamin C
- Vitamin E
- Co enzyme Q10
- Hyaluronic acid
- Ceramides
- Peptides

- Green tea extract
- Dioic acid
- Azelaic acid
- Niacinamide
- Mandelic acid
- Lactic acid

However, complex formulations like this don't exist so I made myself a pregnancy-safe routine with:

1. An anti-melasma exfoliant.
2. An antioxidant, anti-ageing, tyrosinase-inhibiting, pregnancy safe serum using the ingredients above.

Something complex and expensive like this doesn't tend to get made for mass market as it is difficult to make and costs about three times the manufacturing costs of other 'anti-ageing' or 'anti-melasma' products. This makes it unmarketable.

Manufacturers tend to ask the question, 'what is the minimum I can put into a product to market and sell it?'. Any additional ingredient won't translate into more sales and will directly eat into their profit.

The reason I want you to know this is because for you to be truly empowered with your skincare, you need to understand how the manufacturer thinks.

The cosmetic formulator is often working under the direct orders of the factory owner who have price sensitive clients. It is extremely rare for the cosmetic formulator to own the factory and the skincare brand.

The reason I decided to add this to the book is because I hope that cosmetic formulators and consumers will read this and change will happen.

Routine for pregnancy skincare

☀ AM ROUTINE

Step 1: Wash with a micellar gel wash.

Step 2: Moisturise with ceramides and/or peptides.

Step 3: Apply mineral SPF50 as this does not enter bloodstream.

Step 4: Don't forget your wide-brimmed hat and anti-melasma sunglasses to avoid direct UV rays.

☾ PM ROUTINE

Step 1: Wash the face with a simple micellar gel wash.

Step 2: Tone with salicylic acid.

Step 3: Apply niacinamide to improve the skin texture and brighten skin.

Step 4: Apply an antioxidant serum without vitamin A.

Step 5: Finish with a moisturiser with glycerine, sodium hyaluronate, ceramides and cholesterol to increase skin hydration.

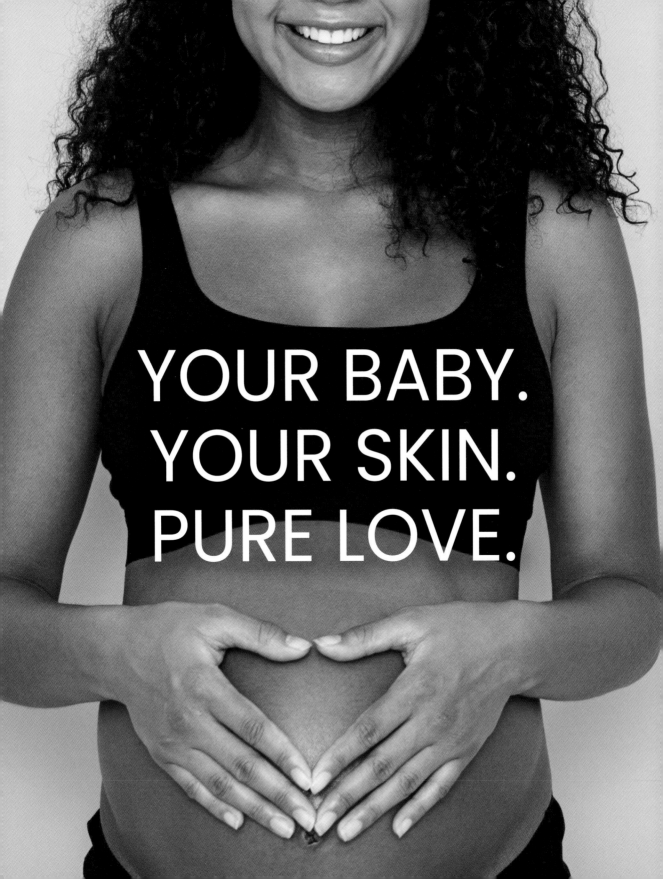

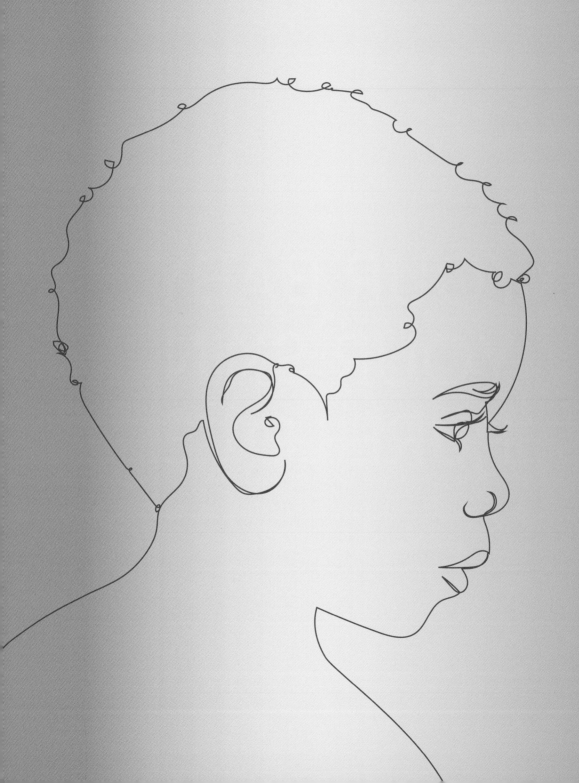

12

Baby, kids and teens
SKINCARE

Babies and young children

Just as they know how to brush their teeth, they should know how to wash their face, dot the moisturiser and apply their sunscreen.

As a parent I wanted my children to feel a sense of independence with their skincare routine. My son is now four years old and has learnt that if he dots the cream I will give him a face massage rubbing the cream in – I can't resist that cherub face!

As a rule of thumb, until 10 years old, a simple three-step routine is all that is needed.

Gentle cleanser

The biggest mistake I see here are heavily fragranced cleansers. Babies or children who bathe will sit in high fragrance for a while. I remember buying my son a 'gentle, baby friendly' bath wash that was marketed as being natural and organic. So in my haste I purchased it, not reading the ingredients. My son got very dry, rough skin after one bathtime and I realised fragrance was very high on the ingredients list. It was my own fault for not checking. Children's skin is more sensitive and doesn't hold water as well as adult skin, which is why we need to minimise stripping oils from their skin or use irritating ingredients.

Great ingredients to look for in children's bath or shampoo products:

Decyl glucoside
Lauryl glucoside
COCO glucoside
Cocamidopropyl betaine
Capryl or capramidopropyl betaine
Disodium laureth sulfosuccinate
Sodium cocyl isethionate

Look for the following humectants and emollients, too:

Triglycerides
Hemp oil
Macadamia oil
Shea butter esters
Humectants, such as panthenol, betaine and glycerine
Prebiotics, such as Inulin

Moisturiser

All soaps can lead to removal of natural skin oils, which is why you must moisturise. In addition, this is a leave-on product so please look at the back of packaging for:

Fragrance
Denatured alcohol
Essential oils

Remember, 'NAFE is SAFE' for my skin-of-colour family

No
Alcohol (denatured)
Fragrance
Essential oils

Please read chapter three on ingredients to avoid as often companies will write the international name of a particular fragrance and you may not recognise it as fragrance.

Moisturise when your child's skin is still a little damp. My kids actually prefer it when I lock in the moisture with an oil that I warm up in my palms.

Oils I use:

Hemp   Grape
Almond

Avoid fragrant oils:

Lavender   Lemon
Rose   Jasmine
Peppermint   Orange

Sunscreen

I am sure you are already using caps and long-sleeve tops when your children are in the water, but don't forget to regularly apply sunscreen.

Please read the chapter on mineral verses chemical sunscreen (see page 66). I tend to recommend mineral sunscreens for children as it doesn't enter the bloodstream. Use a nano-zinc sunscreen to minimise white cast, and which only penetrates the top layer of dead skin cells.

Ingredients to avoid:

Fragrance   Denatured alcohol

So, when do we change our children's routine?

I recommend from about seven years old children should be using a gentle micellar gel wash in the morning – especially if they have a shower or a bath at night.

Pay attention to your children's skin from about 10 years old. If it is becoming oily and congested, switch to the pre-teen skincare routine (see page 259).

What to do when a child has cut their skin

Children are constantly running around jumping off things and cutting or grazing themselves. This is important for their motor functions, speed and spacial awareness. I probably did not do enough of this growing up, which is why it takes me three attempts to park my car!

Unfortunately, a cut often leads to hysterical crying. Dealing with a cut on an adult is bad enough but when the child is grabbing their arm and writhing away from you with large fear-filled eyes and tremor-inducing screams, it is a tad harder.

Step-by-step what to do:

- Stop the bleeding – apply pressure with a clean cloth (avoid tissue, which disintegrates into bits).
- Wash your hands and wash the cut under water to clean any dirt. From experience, this is when the real screaming starts!
- You can apply an antiseptic cream and cover the cut with a non-stick gauze.
- Check the scar daily to ensure it is dry and clean.

Do not scrub or scrape the area and do not use alcohol to clean it. This can lead to further damage and the skin can take longer to heal.

Do not blow on the area, as you are only introducing more germs.

From experience, avoid surgical dressings with very sticky edges. You need to check the scar daily, and often removing the sticky bandage causes more pain than the original cut. Use micropore tape instead, as it is very easy to remove.

Of course, for skin of colour, we worry that cuts on the face may lead to hyperpigmentation. A lot of my fellow school mums are worried about the same thing, so I looked for a tyrosinase-inhibiting cream for children of colour – and it didn't exist! I spoke to my seven-year-old daughter, Sienna, about collaborating with me on this project, and needless to say, she was very excited. We called it Dr V Kids Magic Cream.

Dr V's Formulation Insights

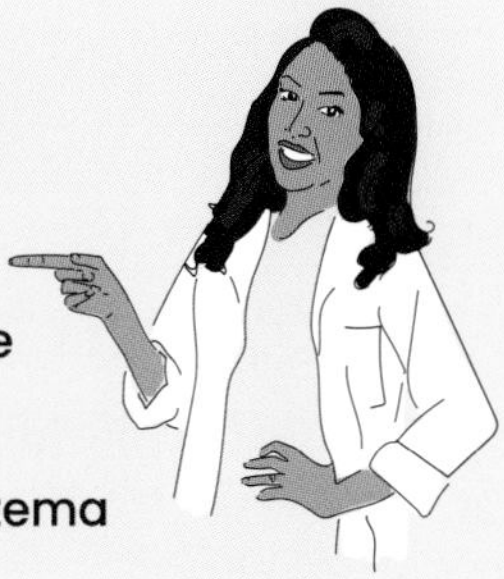

I had never made creams for children before, so I spoke to the assessors to find out what was required.

We had to patch test the Dr V Kids Magic Cream on eczema candidates to see how it reacted.

Ingredients I discovered are safe for children to use after skin has healed are:

Humectants: glycerin, sodium hyaluronate
Emollient/occlusive: jojoba oil, dimethicone, cyclopentasiloxane, shea butter
Anti-inflammatory: panthenol, allantoin
Anti-hyperpigmentation: niacinamide, liquorice root extract, tetrahexyldecyl ascorbate
Antioxidant: tocopheryl acetate

To minimise scarring:

- Apply a kids-safe tyrosinase-inhibiting cream to reduce hyperpigmentation.
- Apply some SPF50 on the area.
- Use silicone gel sheets on top of scar cream to improve hydration and allow skin to heal quickly.

When to see a doctor

You need to call the doctor if the cut is more than half an inch thick or has debris or dirt in it, or it is seeping and looks infected, or if it has affected the eyes or cut the cartilage of the nose or ear.

The doctor can close the cut within 24 hours using:

Skin glue
Skin strips
Stitches

Pre-teens to teens

Teenage years are a nightmare on so many levels, and the pre-teens aren't much better. The body is changing rapidly at this point, and nowadays kids have Instagram to compare themselves to other teens as well, which can make them feel even more insecure about the way they look.

I'll share a little about my own growing pains with you. When I was nine years old, I had giant protruding teeth, so whenever I took a bite out of a biscuit the triangular cut-out was distinctively mine! I had braces, upper lip hair and horrendous bushy brows (which seem to be back in fashion now!) until I was 15/16 years old, and I didn't wax my body hair either. Add to this my Punjabi family's propensity to show their love through overfeeding me and you had a recipe for disaster! While I am pretty sure my strict but well-meaning parents had their own covert aims (namely, to make me look as awful as possible so no boy would even look at me and I would focus on my studies!), I now see how much the beauty standards of the time had a crushing impact on my self-worth. It was something I was too embarrassed to vocalise at the time. I think this may be an issue with most teenagers, which is why I want to reveal all my insecurities so it helps others realise they are not alone.

I am able to laugh it off now, but it was eight painful years of feeling unattractive, insecure and not good enough. I channelled those feelings into my education and pushing myself to get into medical school. I think this is where my work obsession to the point of being self-destructive at times has come from – none of which I want for my own children.

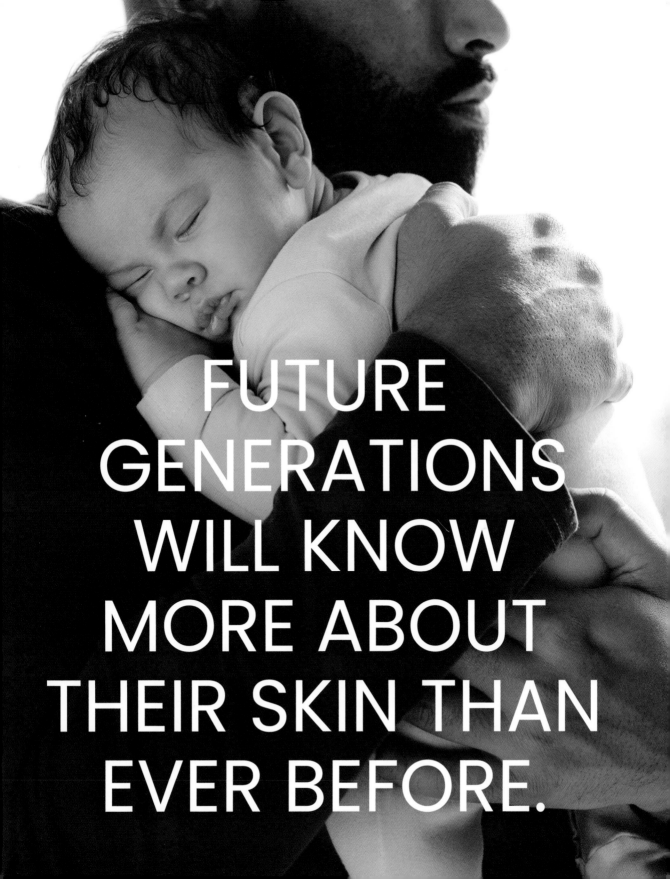

FUTURE GENERATIONS WILL KNOW MORE ABOUT THEIR SKIN THAN EVER BEFORE.

Self-care starts with the way you feel about yourself.

I want to share how I have created stress-releasing, self-love habits that have carried me, and hopefully you too, through the toughest times.

Live for now – remember that you'll never get to relive the moments you're living now, so enjoy them as much as you can. Happiness is essentially contentment. I would fall into the trap of thinking, *'when I pass that exam I'll be happy, when I go to university I will be happy, when I get that car I'll be happy'*. It's possible to spend an entire lifetime this way, only to realise too late that you might have missed the joy that life had to offer.

Build full confidence in yourself – habits and self-limiting beliefs are entrenched in your formative years and can stay with you for life. Building full confidence in yourself in your teenage years allows you to access all the tools you possess already to help you achieve all your dreams and more! Reading Tony Robbins' *Unleash the Power Within* showed me that I can achieve anything I am passionate about. Despite my dyslexia and my English teacher's lack of faith, I wrote this book. I changed my identity from the one that others gave me to my own 'I can do anything, watch me fly'. Remember and believe it – you can do anything you set your mind to.

Nurture stronger relationships with yourself than with others – I was always told that thinking about myself and putting my needs first was selfish, and I know this led to me having to abandon my goals, which was wrong. Now I know we need to 'fill our cup first' and take care of our mental and physical wellbeing before we have the capacity to take care of our loved ones. When we put others first, we neglect ourselves and this leads to unhappiness and resentment. I teach my children to 'check in' with themselves and ask their heart how they feel and what they need to change to feel happy and satisfied. Then you can figure out how to add value to other people's life.

It is essential to also build strong relationships, humans crave connection and loneliness can also affect mental health. Invest time in understanding how you can do this in your own life. One book which helped me was Dale Carnegie's *How to Win Friends and Influence People.* I wish I had read this when I was younger. I specifically decided to create content on TikTok to help the next generation. I know I am definitely NOT cool enough to be on there, but I also know this is an effective way to reach younger people and prevent SkinTok trends from ruining their skin.

As a mum to two beautiful kids, I would never want them to feel insecure or have any of the painful 'not good enough' feelings that I felt growing up. Seeing my babies feel self-conscious even for a second really hurts.

I believe that self-care and self-love comes from small acts of kindness for yourself that reinforce how valuable you are and that you deserve to be loved accordingly – not just now, but for the rest of your life. For me, this includes exercising, eating healthily, meditating, going for long walks listening to my audiobook, scheduled thinking, strategised goal-setting time and my nightly skincare routine.

So, how can we go about creating a skincare routine for our daughters and sons that can become a part of their own routine of self-care and self-acceptance?

First, they need to understand what is happening to their skin.

The increase of hormones in teenagers' bodies during puberty cause the sebaceous glands to enlarge, which increases sebum production (oil production). This excess oil then clogs the pores, which leads to acne – either in the form of white or black heads. (Read chapter six on acne to understand how this works in detail).

Pre-teen to teenage skin

There is no clear time demarcation for when you go from oily, congested skin to full-blown acne. This can happen at different ages and is mainly due to genetics. This is one time you can definitely blame your parents!

If you are a pre-teen with oily congested skin, use this routine:

 AM ROUTINE

Step 1: Cleanse with a soap-free, gentle face wash or micellar gel wash.
Step 2: Apply a non-comedogenic, non-fragranced moisturiser, such as Super gel from Face Theory.
Step 3: Finish off with a non-comedogenic, non-fragranced sunscreen such as Inzincable.

🌙 PM ROUTINE

Step 1: Wash with a salicylic acid face wash, which is oil-soluble to clear out the pores, such as Inkey List.
Step 2: Apply a 2–5% niacinamide serum, such as Naturium or Cerave.
Step 3: Apply a non-comedogenic, non-fragranced moisturiser.

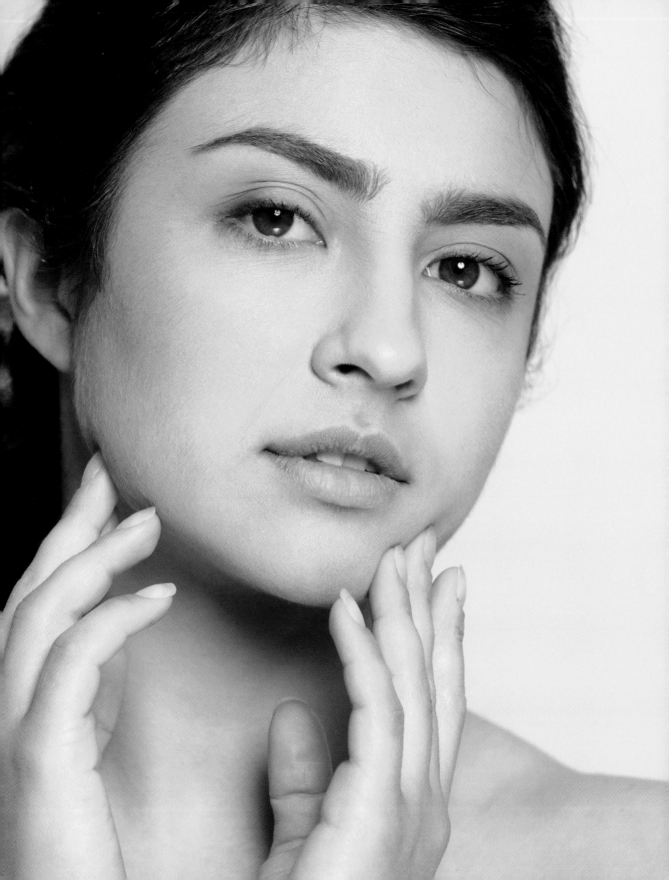

Once you get acne

Use a benzoyl peroxide wash (rather than a salicylic acid wash), leave it on the skin for a minute, then wash it off. This can be drying and your skin is still developing, so you don't want to overuse it and give yourself sensitivity or flaking. If you see this, pause for a couple of days, then try again. Start with washing your face this way on two nights a week for a month. If this is enough, don't do more. In skincare, 'doing more' is not always better for you.

You can then upgrade from salicylic acid wash to 2% salicylic acid leave-on toner (avoid alcohol). If you are starting to get PIE (red marks), add azelaic acid before your niacinamide.

> **When you get a pimple –** cleanse the area with salicylic acid wash, add salicylic acid toner, then use a hydrocolloid patch on top overnight. This will absorb excess sebum from the spot. The following day if I had an important function and the spot looked a little red, I would use 1% hydrocortisone to reduce inflammation. Don't use steroid creams over a long period due to side-effects such as skin thinning.

🌙 EXAMPLE PM ROUTINE:

Step 1: Cleanse with benzoyl peroxide.
Step 2: Apply 2% salicylic acid leave-on product.
Step 3: Apply 2–5% niacinamide serum.
Step 4: Follow up with azelaic acid.
Step 5: Apply a non-comedogenic, non-fragranced moisturiser.

If this is not enough, it is time to see your doctor, who may put you on a vitamin A product.

Inconsistent skincare brings frustration and oily skin. Skin care routines typically yield results after 6-8 weeks of being consistent.

Common mistakes:

Do not scrub the face, as it can worsen acne.

If you are playing sport, take some face wash and a face towel to school. Don't leave sweat on your face.

Ideally, avoid wearing makeup, if you do need to wear makeup, I tend to prefer a mineral powder over a liquid foundation. Eye makeup or lipstick won't worsen acne. Make sure you remove all makeup every night and do not share makeup.

Wash your hands before touching your face and clean your phone if it touches your face.

A common cause of forehead acne is haircare oils and balms seeping onto the face.

Do not apply toothpaste or essential oils to a spot, as they are skin sensitisers, and avoid denatured alcohol as it can dry the skin.

Do not squeeze pimples – this can damage the pore lining and you will get recurrent spots in the same location.

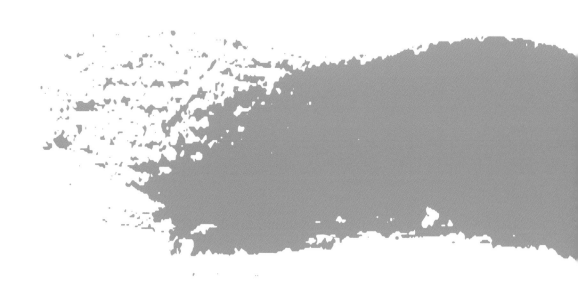

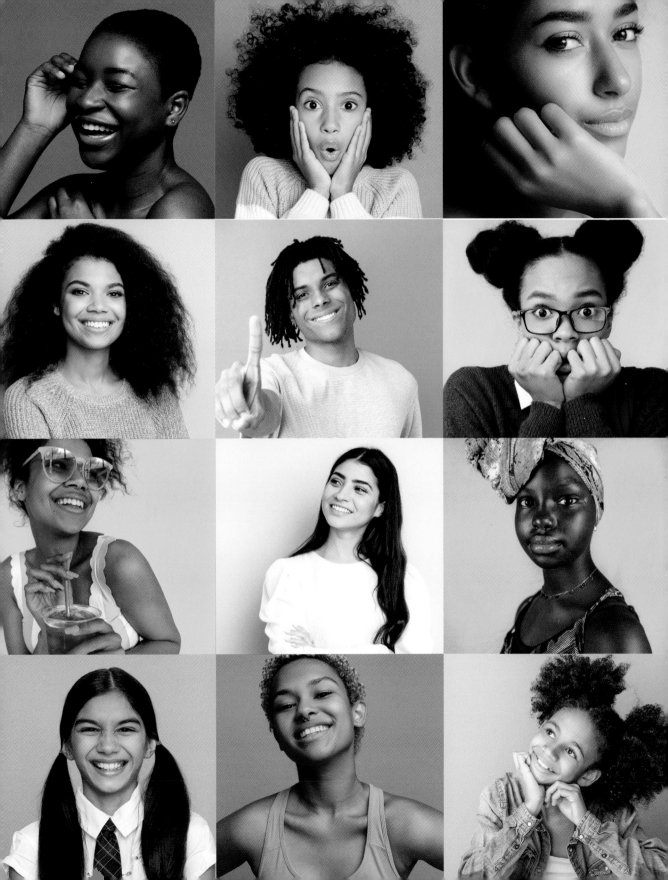

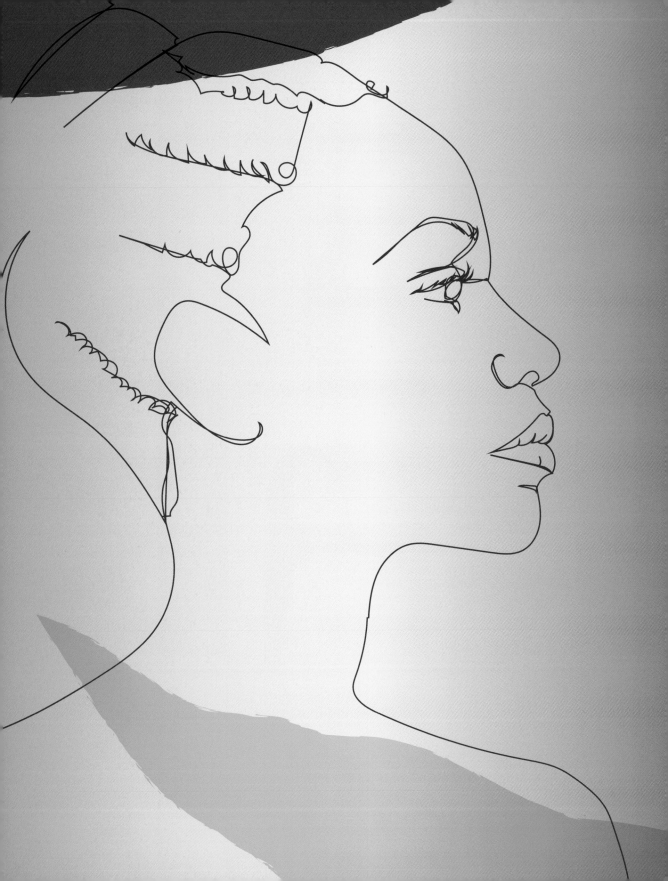

13

SKIN
concern combinations

Often we do not just have one skin condition, we have a combination of different issues, so I want to break it down for you to make sure you know what to look for in your products.

In treating one condition you could make another condition worse.

It can be a minefield understanding the complex needs of your skin. I asked followers of **@SkincarebyDrV** what their skin problem combinations were and I have chosen the most common concerns below.

Melasma + ageing + dullness

These are the main skin issues in my case. Dynamic lines are settling into static lines, this is the downside of having big teeth (I blame my grandad!).

   Melasma started early in my mid-twenties. I remember my first 'freckle' and trying to scratch it off thinking I had just smudged eye liner, but realising that it was in fact early signs of sun damage. It is only when you start to get skin issues that you pay attention to your skin, otherwise we tend to take it for granted.

The aim here is to:

1. Reduce the rate of melanin production.
2. Boost collagen.
3. Exfoliate gently and use skin brightening agents.

Ideal ingredients:

Hyperpigmentation/ melasma	Reduce rate of melanin production	Tyrosinase inhibitors, such as alpha arbutin, octadecanedioic acid, kojic dipalmitate
Ageing	Boost collagen	Tetrahexyldecyl ascorbate (fat-soluble vitamin C), retinol, retinyl palmitate, retinaldehyde, peptides
Dullness	Exfoliate gently	Lactic and mandelic acid
	Brightening agents	Vitamin C, niacinamide
	Humectants	Glycerin, urea

Common mistakes:

Not re-applying SPF50 sunscreen throughout the day to block UV to prevent melasma and premature ageing. It is common not to re-apply because people feel they can't do this over makeup – if this is you, I have made videos on YouTube showing how I re-apply over makeup.

It is also advisable to wear oversized sunglasses and a wide-brimmed hat to prevent direct UV light hitting the face on prominent facial areas (upper cheeks, temples, around the eyes).

Skin becomes drier and more sensitive, especially if you are wearing vitamin A. Ensure you use a fatty, non-fragrance moisturiser before and after you apply the vitamin A product. Keep retinol at less than 0.5% to minimise chances of irritation.

Rather than increasing retinol percentage to improve results I would rather you use all three forms of over-the-counter vitamin A simultaneously so you are at every stage of the vitamin A pathway – i.e. retinyl palmitate, retinol and retinalde-hyde. This is more effective because there is less irritation, which means greater compliance than higher percentages of retinol.

Keep your low-pH acids and vitamin A serums for your nighttime routine.

The other classic mistake is to over exfoliate. This gives temporary brightening but will damage the skin barrier, lead to sensitivity and stop you wearing your tyrosinase-inhibiting creams.

Routine:

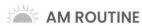 **AM ROUTINE**

Step 1: Wash with gentle micellar gel. If you feel there are actives still on the skin in the morning, you can double cleanse, but don't do this if the skin feels dry as you don't want to over-strip the skin.

Step 2: Use a fatty, non-fragrance moisturiser with ceramides and peptides.

Step 3: Apply SPF50 (I prefer mineral for melasma).

🌙 **PM ROUTINE**

Step 1: Double cleanse (remove makeup and sunscreen).

Step 2: Use a tyrosinase-inhibiting cream on the melasma.

Step 3: Apply anti-ageing vitamin A cream on fine wrinkles and neck (usually I say vitamin A first but here the more pressing issue is melasma over ageing, which is why we want maximum penetration of tyrosinase inhibitors).

Step 4: Use a fatty non-fragrance moisturiser with ceramides and peptides.

Ageing + acne + hyperpigmentation

This is a tricky one as quite a few different actives are needed. It would be wise to use actives with multiple benefits – such as vitamin A, which is anti-ageing, helps with acne and improves pigmentation. Azelaic acid is another ingredient that helps with acne, red marks from acne and hyperpigmentation. Niacinamide also assists with sebum control and hyperpigmentation.

Aim:

Boost collagen production
Reduce acne breakouts
Reduce hyperpigmentation

Ideal ingredients:

Anti-ageing	Boost collagen production	Tetrahexyldecyl ascorbate (fat-soluble vitamin C), retinol, retinyl palmitate, retinaldehyde, peptides
Reduce acne breakouts	Control sebum production	Niacinamide
	Unclog pores	Salicylic acid
	Kill C. acnes	Benzoyl peroxide
Reduce hyper-pigmentation	Reduce rate of melanin production	Tyrosinase inhibitors, such as alpha arbutin, azelaic acid, octadecanedioic acid, kojic dipalmitate

Common mistakes:

Over-doing benzoyl peroxide – please stick with 2.5% to avoid excessive flaking, irritation and sensitivity. Please only apply benzoyl peroxide on the actual spots, not the whole face, as you have actives that need to go on other areas.

Always wait until the benzoyl peroxide has dried before applying your anti-oxidant products. Don't forget that benzoyl peroxide is essentially poisoning C. acnes bacteria with oxygen, so you want this action to complete before you apply an antioxidant or it won't be effective.

I would focus your tyrosinase-inhibiting creams on the actual pigmentation, benzoyl peroxide on the active spots and anti-ageing products on the fine lines. I tend to derma-roll my own static lines and add my anti-ageing serum to make sure I am getting the product into the correct location without unnecessarily irritating the rest of the skin. I also focus my anti-ageing products on my neck as this will age quickly.

As before, the other mistake I see is people not being obsessive enough with their SPF50. No amount of vitamin A will work if you are not re-applying your SPF50 every few hours. Some people get confused, thinking tanning will make hyperpigmentation fade, but this is a mistake as all you are doing is camouflaging the pigmentation by making the surrounding skin darker, but once your skin has lost its tan, the hyperpigmentation may appear even darker and UVA has further aged the skin.

Routine:

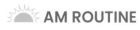 **AM ROUTINE**

Step 1: Wash with salicylic acid wash.

Step 2: Apply a non-comedogenic, fragrance-free, denatured alcohol-free gel moisturiser.

Step 3: Use SPF50 (I prefer mineral for hyperpigmentation for inflamed skin).

🌙 **PM ROUTINE**

Step 1: Remove makeup with micellar water.

Step 2: Wash with benzoyl peroxide or salicylic acid wash then apply benzoyl peroxide cream to the spots.

Step 3: Use a tyrosinase-inhibiting cream on the melasma.

Step 4: Apply an anti-ageing vitamin A cream on fine wrinkles and the neck.

Step 5: Non-comedogenic, fragrance-free, denatured alcohol-free gel moisturiser.

Hyperpigmentation + combination skin + clogged pores

This is very common and clogged pores can happen the week before menstruation (period). The key actives you want to use are salicylic acid, niacinamide and tyrosinase inhibitors. It is a fairly easy routine.

Aim:

- Reduce hyperpigmentation.
- Control the oil on the T-zone and hydrate drier cheeks.
- Unclog pores and minimise their appearance.

Ideal ingredients:

Hyperpigmentation	Reduce rate of melanin production	Tyrosinase inhibitors, such as alpha arbutin, octadecanedioic acid, kojic dipalmitate, liquorice root, bearberry extract
Combination skin	Control oil on T-zone	Niacinamide on forehead and nose, lighter moisturiser
	Hydrate drier cheeks	Heavier, more emollient moisturiser on cheeks
Pores	Unclog pores and minimise the appearance	Salicylic acid

Routine:

 ## AM ROUTINE

Step 1: Wash with a gentle micellar gel wash. Potentially, use a salicylic acid wash on the T-zone.
Step 2: Apply a fatty non-fragrance moisturiser to the cheeks and a gel moisturiser to the T-zone
Step 3: Finish with SPF50.

 ## PM ROUTINE

Step 1: Double cleanse (remove makeup and sunscreen).
Step 2: Use a tyrosinase-inhibiting cream on hyperpigmentation.
Step 3: Apply azelaic acid and niacinamide on T-zone.
Step 4: Finish with a fatty non-fragrance moisturiser with ceramides and peptides on cheeks and gel moisturiser for T-zone.

Dry skin + eczema + wrinkles

By definition, eczema means a damaged skin barrier and increased water loss from the skin, leading to dry, dehydrated skin and often premature wrinkles. The issue here is that most anti-ageing products contain vitamin A, which can further dry the skin. I do NOT recommend this.

Aim:

• To hydrate the skin and use non-irritating ingredients once skin barrier has recovered.
• Hydrate the skin to plump the top layer of skin so light bounces off it evenly.
• Do NOT irritate the skin, as this will lead to a flare up.

Ideal ingredients:

Anti-ageing	Boost collagen production, strengthen skin barrier	peptides, ceramides
Smooth wrinkles	Hydrate	Humectants, such as hyaluronic acid, glycerine, urea
	Reduce water evaporation	Petrolatum, paraffinum
Anti- inflammatory	Soothe skin	Aloe, panthenol

Common mistakes:

Avoid all low-pH acids, fragrance, denatured alcohol, essential oils, vitamin A.

Sunscreen is key here more than ever. UVA is the number one cause of premature ageing. Keep both your thick heavy emollient and SPF50 (I prefer mineral for inflammed skin) in your bag at all times.

Be aware of the triggers, including stress, drop in temperature, hot showers or baths, detergents with fragrance, dust mites, pet dander, drinking alcohol or excessive sweating.

Avoid makeup on eczema-inflamed skin.

Routine:

 ## AM ROUTINE

Step 1: Avoid washing the face in the morning if the skin feels dry.
Step 2: Apply a fatty, soothing, non-fragrance moisturiser with ceramides and peptides.
Step 3: Apply SPF50 (I prefer mineral).

 ## PM ROUTINE

Step 1: Wash with gentle micellar gel then rinse quickly with lukewarm water.
Step 2: Apply a fatty, soothing, non-fragrance moisturiser with ceramides and peptides.

Cystic acne + hyperpigmentation + sensitive skin

Cystic acne means you need to visit your dermatologist, as a sudden loss of collagen from a cyst rupturing can lead to scarring, which is incredibly difficult to treat.

I won't write a routine on this as you may be on 'Roaccutane', in which case you don't want to be applying any other actives.

Aim:

- Reduce oily skin.
- Kill C.acnes bacteria.
- Reduce hyperpigmentation using tyrsoinase inhibitors.
- Ensure skin barrier is intact.

Common mistakes:

I have seen teenagers scrub their skin to try to remove the oil slick, which damages the skin barrier and leads to redness, flaking and sensitivity to actives.

Avoid stripping alcohol toners, this squeaky clean feeling is temporary and you are likely to get more oily skin. Don't try to treat this at home.

Dark spots + fine lines + dark circles

The epidermis on the cheek is thicker than under the eyes, so you need different strength actives for hyperpigmentation on the cheeks and for around the eyes. For example, I am happy for you to use mandelic acid or lactic acid for the cheeks, but I wouldn't advise this for under the eyes.

Aim:

- Reduce hyperpigmentation on face.
- Reduce periorbital pigmentation.
- Reduce the appearance of fine lines.

Ideal ingredients:

Face pigmentation	Acids and tyrosinase inhibitors	Mandelic acid, lactic acid (plus the tyrosinase-inhibiting chapter)
Periorbital pigmentation	Gentle tyrosinase inhibitors	Niacinamide, kojic dipalmitate, alpha arbutin, octadecenedioic acid, liquorice root extract
Fine lines	Humectants and collagen boosters	Peptides, ceramides, tetrahexyl decylascorbate, hyaluronic acid, glycerine

All the tyrosinase inhibitors for around the eye area are suitable for the face too.

Common mistakes:

I have seen people peel the periorbital area, which leads to temporary results at best, but the downside is that this skin is already 0.3mm thin, so we need to stimulate collagen and 'thicken' the skin, not peel it.

I have also seen the importance of sunscreen underestimated. UVA rays worsen pigmentation and this leads to premature ageing. You need a broad-spectrum SPF50.

Uneven texture + dry skin + milia

The uneven texture is usually due to acne scarring.

Aim:

There are limited solutions to this. Micro-needling is one of them, to break up collagen and allow new 'normal' lattice collagen to be formed. You shouldn't do this if your skin is sensitive or dry. You first want to ensure skin is hydrated, creating a 'healing' environment for the skin. Milia tend to need a professional to remove them.

Ideal ingredients:

Uneven texture	Repair collagen	Peptides, tetrahexyldecylascorbate, vitamin A (Retinyl palmitate, retinaldehyde, retinol)
	Exfoliate	Lactic acid, mandelic acid
Dry skin	Humectants and occlusives	Peptides, ceramides, tetrahexyl decyl ascorbate, hyaluronic acid, glycerine

Broken, irritated skin + acne + post-acne pigmentation

The issue here is that is the skin barrier is damaged, you cannot then use strong actives, such as benzoyl peroxide.

Aim:

You must first repair the skin barrier. Once the barrier is hydrated and strong you can start slowly spot-treating with benzoyl peroxide and salicylic acid. Use gentle actives for pigmentation such as azelaic acid, niacinamide and alpha arbutin.

Ideal ingredients:

Please read the acne and post-acne pigmentation chapter from page 171.

Common mistakes:

People sometimes feel that if the skin is 'tingling' and 'burning' the product is working, but actually the opposite is true, especially for skin of colour. We should not experience any burning with cosmetic products. If you do, please stop straight away and seek advice.

The Ultimate Skincare Glossary

Acanthosis nigricans: Brown, velvety patches in folds of body, such as the neck, groin or armpits.

Acid mantle: Slightly acidic pH 4.5–6 thin film on skin acting as the first barrier or defence against pathogens. Composed of fats and amino acids and sweat.

Actives: Skincare ingredients with a specific temporary action on skin cells.

Antioxidant: Substance that neutralises damaging free radicals. Free radicals oxidise cells leading to premature ageing and worsening of active skin conditions.

Astringent: Removes oil from the skin.

Basal layer: Base of epidermis, where skin cells are manufactured (keratinocytes) and where cells that produce melanin live (melanocytes).

C. acnes: Cutibacterium acnes grows in oxygen-deprived sebaceous glands, leading to acne.

Capillary: Small blood vessels that allow exchange of substances between blood and surrounding tissue, such as oxygen.

Ceramides: Naturally occurring fats found in the skin between skin cells. They prevent water loss from the skin.

Chromphores: In skin, a chromophore absorbs visible light. The main chromophores of human skin are haemoglobin and melanin.

Collagen: Most abundant protein in the body. Found in skin, bones and muscles.

Comedogenic: A product that clogs pores and leads to white heads.

Dandruff: Flaky, itchy scalp, often visible as white flakes on shoulders.

Dermaplaning: Exfoliating blade that removes dead skin cells and vellus hair on the face.

Dermatitis: Inflammation of skin. It can look red, swollen, dry and flaky.

Dermis: Skin layer deeper than the epidermis. Contains hair follicles, blood vessels, oil and sweat glands and nerves.

Eczema, aka Atopic Dermatitis: Inflammation of skin seen as dry, cracked, flaky skin, which may bleed.

Elastin: Protein found in skin that allows skin to stretch and snap back to its original position.

Emollient: Skincare ingredients that soften and smooth skin cells, used for dry skin.

Enzyme: Controls rate of a chemical reaction.

Epidermis: Top layer of skin protecting from micro-organisms and giving us our skin colour.

Erythema: Red or burgundy colour of skin as a result of infection, inflammation or irritation.

Fatty acid: Used in skincare as an emollient or to hydrate. Free fatty acids are formed from C. acnes, however, are irritating, leading to acne inflammation.

Fibroblast: Cells that produce collagen.

Fitzpatrick Scale: Classification of skin colour according to how it responds to UV light. Skin of colour is considered to be 4–6.

Free radical: When an atom in skin contains one or more unpaired electrons. They are highly reactive and unstable. They damage collagen in skin, leading to premature ageing.

Fungus: Fungal infections tend to occur in moist warm areas of the body. The most common are yeast Candida or Malassezia.

Glucosaminoglycans: Highly polar molecules that attract water. The common one is hyaluronic acid.

Glycation: Sugar irreversibly attaches to proteins including collagen and elastin. This leads to ageing of the skin.

Humectant: Ingredients that behave like a water magnet, such as urea, hyaluronic acid and glycerin.

Hyperpigmentation: Dark patches seen on skin from overactive melanocytes (melanin-producing cells). Cells may be triggered by inflammation, irritation or UV radiation.

Hypoallergenic: Unregulated term. Assumes product produces fewer reactions than average.

Hypogpigmentation: Reduction in pigmentation, seen as white or lighter patches on the skin.

Keloid: Excess growth of scar tissue outside the original site of trauma.

Keratinocytes: Main skin cell found in the epidermis.

Keratosis Pilaris, aka 'chicken skin': Keratin plugging the hair follicle leading to rough, bumpy skin.

Lipid: Natural fats found in skin that retain moisture and keep micro-organisms out.

Lipophilic: Literally means lipid-loving. It is the affiliation to fats such as salicylic acid.

Malassezia: Yeast found on skin that can lead to fungal acne or seborrheic dermatitis.

Melanin: Pigment found in skin, hair and eyes.

Melanocyte: Cell that produces the pigment melanin.

Melanogenesis: The production of melanin.

Melasma: Brown facial pigmentation primarily in females from the twenties onwards. Usually occurs on cheek bones, forehead and upper lip.

Micelle: A ball of surfactant molecules with water-loving ends in the solvent and fat-loving ends in the center of the micelle.

Moisture barrier: Prevents transepidermal water loss (TEWL) and keeps skin hydrated.

Niacinamide: Vitamin B3, excellent skincare ingredient for sebum control, pigmentation and erythema.

Non-comedogenic: Non-pore clogging product.

Occlusive: Skincare ingredient forming a film on the skin that prevents water loss, essential in a moisturiser.

Oxidise: When a compound loses an electron. This happens when sebum in pores oxidises and lead to black heads or when antioxidants oxidise in air then become ineffective in skincare.

P. acne: Shortened form of Propionibacterium acnes, the main bacteria responsible for acne.

Pathology: The cause of a disease and how it develops.

Peptides: Chain of 2–50 amino acids needed for hydration and improved skin texture in skincare.

PIE: Post-inflammatory Erythema – red marks seen after trauma, such as after acne.

pH: Measure of acid or alkali solution.

PIH: Post-inflammatory Hyperpigmentation. Brown marks seen after trauma such as an insect bite, cut, scar or acne.

Pore: Small opening on the skin above the hair follicle. Sebum is released onto the skin via pores.

Psoriasis: A skin condition leading to red scaly patches on the skin.

Razor burn: When shaving leads to irritation and inflammation.

Rosacea: Skin condition leading to flare ups of redness, sensitivity, broken capillaries on the cheeks and nose.

Seborrheic dermatitis: Malassezia yeast overgrowth leading to inflammation of skin and in turn to red, scaly, flaky skin on the scalp and face.

Sebum: Mixture of fatty acids, wax esters and squalene secreted from the sebaceous gland to prevent water evaporation from skin.

Skin barrier: Physical barrier keeping microorganisms out.

Soluble: An ingredient is able to dissolve in water if water-soluble or in oil if oil-soluble.

Solvent: Liquid used to dissolve a substance to make a solution.

SPF: Sun Protection Factor. Applies to UVB rays.

Stratum corneum: Outer layer of dead skin cells.

Surfactants: Ingredient used to reduce surface tension of solvent and improve wetting ability or spreadability.

TEWL: Transepidermal Water Loss (water evaporation from skin).

Tyrosinase inhibitor: Ingredients used to treat hyperpigmentation by slowing the enzyme Tyrosinase.

UVA: Part of the electromagnetic spectrum that leads to ageing. This is why you want a broad-spectrum sunscreen (320 to 400 nm).

UVB: Part of the electromagnetic spectrum that leads to burning of the skin. This is why you want an SPF50 sunscreen (280 to 320 nm).

Vasoconstriction: Narrowing of the blood vessels.

Vasodilation: Expansion of the blood vessels, this occurs during inflammation, which leads to heat and redness.

Index

Page references in *italics* indicate images.

A

Acanthosis nigricans 139, 206–7, 276

acid mantle 24, 52, 181, 276

acids 90–5

acne 25, 109, 111, 144, 152, 156, 166–95, 201, 207, 220, 221, 222, 230, 233, 234, 237, 259, 261, 262, 268, 274, 276, 277, 278; actives and 52; back 185–6; bacteria and 176–83; categories 177; causes 170–5; combinations, skin concern 268–70, 275; cystic 184, 273; dry skin with 192–5; hormonal 189–91; hypopigmentation and 184; *Malassezia folliculitis* (fungal acne) 187–8; mistakes 175, 184

actives 50–3

aftershave 228, 229, 231, 232, 237

ageing 21, 22, 23, 37, 38, 41, 42, 44, 49, 50, 52, 56, 58, 62, 66, 67, 70, 76, 81, 85, 86, 87, 92, 94, 96, 129, 141, 148, 149, 150, 189, 192, 220, 221, 228, 229, 232, 276, 277, 278; actives and 52; anti-ageing step-by-step routine 153; anti-ageing, pregnancy skincare routine 246; anti-ageing term 35; combinations, skin concern 266–70; decades, skincare through the 155–64; premature, risk of free radicals and 150–2; skin and 148–50

alcohol 14, 31, 40, 42, 49, 74, 84, 93, 103, 129, 137, 142, 150, 151, 153, 175, 184, 186, 192, 194, 195, 200, 201, 209, 221, 229, 231, 232, 234, 236, 237, 253, 254, 261, 262, 270, 272, 273; denatured 14, 38, 40, 45, 46, 93, 96, 105, 109, 112, 142, 184, 186, 192, 194, 195, 200, 212, 229, 231, 237, 253, 254, 262, 270, 272; drying 29, 103, 153, 205; in skincare 95–6; toners and 38, 45, 46, 57, 65, 109

alkyl surfactant 43–4, *43*

alpha hydroxy acids (AHA) 29, 41, 48, 92, 94, 109, 113, 118, 125, 140, 149, 163, 185, 195, 223, 246; vs BHA 47–8, *47*; glycolic acid *see* glycolic acid

amino acids (peptides) 29, 30, 35, 46, 50, 52, 53, 58, 62, 89, 93, 94, 97, 99, 149, 152, 153, 160, 161, 153, 195, 221, 230, 246, 247, 248, 267, 268, 269, 271, 272, 274, 276, 277

animal testing 34

antioxidants 26, 35, 37, 45, 46, 50, 51, 52, 58, 64, 71, 76, 83, 87, 89, 95, 97, 99, 107, 109, 122, 128, 129, 133, 135, 136, 150, 151, 153, 155, 156, 158, 160, 161, 162, 163, 164, 181, 182, 229, 230, 231, 232, 237, 245, 247, 248, 255, 269, 276, 277

ascorbic acid 71, 81, 86, 88, 89, 90, 93, 94, 106–7, 122, 135, 181

astringent 40, 276

azelaic acid 38, 50, 52, 95, 122, 129, 132, 135, 173, 181, 245, 247, 261, 268, 269, 271, 275

B

babies and young children 252–6

basal layer 21, *21*, 22, 23, 206, 276

benzoyl peroxide 44, 50, 52, 83, 107, 109, 111, 155, 156, 172, 173, 174, 186, 188, 191, 192, 193, 220, 233, 261, 269, 270, 275

beta hydroxy acid (BHA) 48, 90, 47–8

breakouts 26, 111

C

C. acnes 95, 173, 176, 178, 185, 193, 222, 269, 273, 276

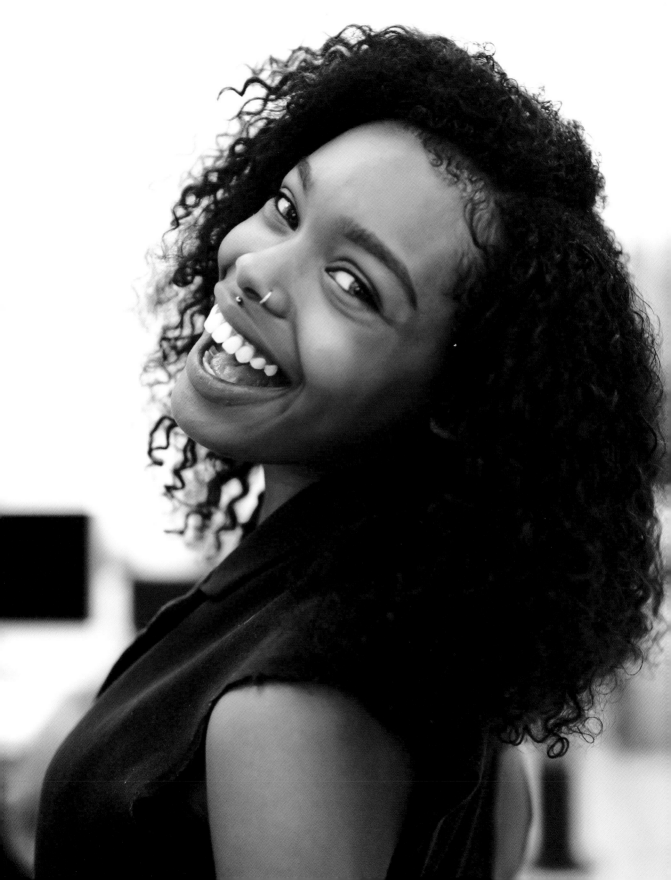

Acknowledgements

I warn you now, I am beyond grateful to a long list of incredible people ... hold on to your seats!

My husband, my whole world. I thank god every day I found you. I keep reaching higher and pushing harder and you give me all the support I need to touch the stars. Your belief in me and staking your life on me shakes my core, thank you for being the world's greatest husband. You were also the gateway for me to meet my Rattan family who I have felt were my own from day one.

My daughter and son, Sienna and Josh. I never knew what it was to cry with happiness until you were born. I am so grateful to be your mother and I am so proud of you both. I love your confidence starting your own YouTube channel. I love your work ethic Sisi and I loved collaborating with you on the Dr V Kids Magic Cream. Josh, you just charm your way though life, may that never end.

To my parents, I wouldn't have had the education or the strength to achieve any of my goals without you. Thank you for having high expectations of me and pushing me past my limits.

To the whole Rattan Clan, I am one of the lucky few to have the best in laws ever! I receive unconditional love and support, thank you for being you.

My brother Shiv, you are a super star. Thank you for always having my back and supporting all my decisions even if they were unpopular, I can never repay you for being my rock. You seem to know exactly what to say to get me back on track and help me strive for more. Esha, my gorgeous and kind sister-in-law, we were blessed when you entered our home.

My dearest Seema Aunty who I dedicate this book to. You were the happiness in my childhood, I can still hear you say 'Vimtooo is here! Let's go swimming and Pizza Hut!' and you trained me to always introduce you as my 'favourite aunty' which was genius! You were taken too soon from us but I promise your light lives in us all. You taught us contentment and forgiveness. I love you and miss you.

Shivani my TikTok superstar director and my now not so secret weapon!

To my big beautiful Punjabi family, who love hard and live loud from my grandparents, aunties and uncles to Pranav, Shefali, Varun, Anisha, Ravina, Avinash, Prab, Nikhita, Aman, Saahil and Sonika – love you all.

Noureen, you convinced me I was good enough to start an Instagram channel. You literally shot all my content for a year and to this day are my well of confidence. God really did bless me with you. Thank you.

Camille, you are my right and left hand. Thank you for being so incredible. You literally typed out this book from my scrawly handwriting, manage all our social media, show me my blind spots and most important keep my mind cool when I become overwhelmed. I couldn't do any of this without you! Thank you, Thank you.

Amandeep, you are the best editor I could have asked for. I was terrified starting this project but you put me at ease and held my hand through it all. Thank you for making this dream come true for me.

Paulina, you are such an incredible formulator and teacher, when we started this journey years ago over Whatsapp trying to build a laboratory in the UK, it felt nearly impossible but you are super woman and can make anything happen. Thank you for trusting me and being with me every step of the way. Kaisa, you are one hard working lady. None of this would be possible without you.

Thank you Emma and Stephen for taking all the stress of manufacturing from me. You made this all possible, people like you are rare and I value you. Thank you!

Lorna and Sarah you were incredible on the Inzincable™ project and I am so grateful for your contribution to the sunscreen chapter.

Thankyou Dr Ravinder Atkar for your diligent fact checking and for your huge contribution to the acne and eczema chapters. This book would not have been the same without you.

My agent Jane from Graham Maw Christie and Vex King – thank you Vex for believing in me and introducing me to Jane, none of this would have been possible without you. There are some special people in the world who honestly want the best for you and hand on heart this applies to you both, thank you.

Omer and Anisha for the epic photo shoot for this book and our skincare campaigns.

Moving onto my friends who are more like family!

We have shared happy times, sad times and lived our dreams together since university 20 years ago. Shaz, Sheena, Visheena, Deepa, Sheetal, Aketa, Nisa, Chandini, Sonia, Gopal, Sarika and Sheetal. I love that I can rely on you till this day, how did I get so lucky?

To my amazing mummy friends Manisha, Shikha, Shrijal, Divi, Raj, Nisha, Swita, Sonia, Sonali, Melissa, Subina, Sue, Shamyka, Arti, Anjani, Nutan, Lakshmi, Seema and Reena. You don't usually think in your 30s you will find such an incredible group of supportive ladies but then you came along and proved me wrong. I love that our babies are growing up together. Love you ladies! Now I get to meet a whole new set of incredible and inspiring mums from Josh's new school! Thank you ladies for your feedback on all my future products!

Thank you Sarah for all your stunning design work for my social media and products, we couldn't move at this speed without you.

Thank you Sapna from Phoenix, you always come through for me on any emergency ingredients. I am so grateful for you!

Thank you Eileen for believing in me from such a young age. I really feel that when you tell a child they are capable of anything they will believe they can move mountains. Self belief was the greatest gift you could have given me, thank you.

Thank you HarperCollins for believing in me and my vision for our skin-of-colour family, you made us feel seen and I will be eternally grateful for this opportunity, I hope I can make you proud!

About the author

Dr Vanita Rattan is a cosmetic formulator specialising in skin of colour and a doctor in Medicine (MBBS) and Physiology/Pharmacology (BSc). In 2012 she started her cosmetic formulator training, where after five painstaking years she pioneered the world's first professional grade pigmentation treatment for skin of colour. Dr Vanita has treated over 40,000 cases of hyperpigmentation globally with a 95 per cent success rate. She was also awarded a 2009 BMA Book Award for outstanding contribution to medical literature. Dr Vanita has grown her social media platform by over a million followers as she continues to provide non-sponsored teaching for the global skin of colour community. She owns her own laboratory to conduct research and development on ingredients, percentages and combinations suitable for skin of colour. Her goal is to ensure equal skincare practices for skin of colour as for Caucasian skin, which she believes will come from education and empowerment.

@drvanitarattan @skincarebydrv @drvanitarattan
Dr. Vanita Rattan The Hyperpigmentation Clinic
www.skincarebydrv.com

Endnotes

1. Proksch E, Segger D, Degwert J, Schunck M, Zague V, Oesser S. Oral supplementation of specific collagen peptides has beneficial effects on human skin physiology: a double-blind, placebo-controlled study. Skin Pharmacol Physiol. 2014;27(1):47-55. doi: 10.1159/000351376. Epub 2013 Aug 14. PMID: 23949208.

2. Oliver, B., Krishnan, S., Rengifo Pardo, M. et al. Cosmeceutical Contact Dermatitis— Cautions To Herbals. Curr Treat Options Allergy 2, 307–321 (2015).

3. Davis, Erica C, and Valerie D Callender. Postinflammatory hyperpigmentation: a review of the epidemiology, clinical features, and treatment options in skin of color. The Journal of clinical and aesthetic dermatology vol. 3,7 (2010): 20-31.

4. Pittayapruek, Pavida et al. 'Role of Matrix Metalloproteinases in Photoaging and Photocarcinogenesis.' International journal of molecular sciences vol. 17,6 868. 2 Jun. 2016, doi:10.3390/ijms17060868.

5. Zari, Shadi, and Dana Alrahmani. "The association between stress and acne among female medical students in Jeddah, Saudi Arabia." Clinical, cosmetic and investigational dermatology vol. 10 503-506. 5 Dec. 2017, doi:10.2147/CCID.S148499.

6. M.K. Trivedi, G. Kroumpouzos, J.E. Murase, A review of the safety of cosmetic procedures during pregnancy and lactation, International Journal of Women's Dermatology, Volume 3, Issue 1, 2017, Pages 6-10, ISSN 2352-6475, https://doi.org/10.1016/j.ijwd.2017.01.005.